BISHOP'S BREW

To Elizabeth, Robert, and Nicholas,
Grandchildren,
For the laughter and the joy they
have brought.

BISHOP'S BREW

An Anthology of Clerical Humour

Compiled by

RONALD BROWN

Bishop of Birkenhead

Arthur James

BOOK PUBLISHERS

BISHOP'S BREW
By
Ronald Brown
First published in hardback by
Churchman Publishing Limited, 1989
First published in paperback in 1991 by
ARTHUR JAMES Limited
One Cranbourne Road, London N10 2BT
Great Britain

© Ronald Brown
World rights reserved by the publishers,
Arthur James Limited

British Library Cataloguing in Publication Data

Brown, Ronald, *1926—*
Bishop's brew.
I. Title
827.91408

ISBN 0 85305 317 0

Printed by
The Guernsey Press Co. Ltd, Guernsey, Channel Islands

FOREWORD

ALL ROYALTIES from the sale of this book will go to the Church Urban Fund which has been set up by the Archbishop of Canterbury to assist the work of the Church in difficult and deprived areas of the country.

To my own collection of stories gathered over many years I have added about as many again from those sent me by past and present members of the clergy of the Chester Diocese. I am most grateful to them all and rejoice in the fellowship and happiness we have together in the gospel of Jesus Christ.

My gratitude also goes to the Reverend Graeme Skinner, an assistant curate in the Chester Diocese, for the illustrations: and to Mr. Roger Barley for his invaluable help in the typing and sorting of the material.

Truth really is sometimes stranger than fiction and not a few of the anecdotes are said to be true or based on fact. I leave it to the reader to make a judgement in this respect. There is certainly a wide variety in the type of things that amuse which I hope is reflected in the pages that follow. The one thing I hope is missing is anything that causes hurt or gives offence to anyone.

Not everything in the book is new, of course, though there is, I believe, a pleasing amount of original material. I think it is good to have in a collection of this kind things old and new from the treasury of church humour. This is a reminder that at all times and in all ages we should not take ourselves too seriously for our trust lies beyond this world and its foibles.

What a special and valuable gift humour is, for as we all know it can ease the heavy burden, deepen fellowship, and reveal human frailty, but like all God's gifts it is here to be used and enjoyed rather than analysed, yet another example of His wisdom and love. If I thought that even a faint whisper of this could be detected in these pages I would have cause for rejoicing.

'Bring laughter to thy great employ,
Go forth with God and find His joy.'

+RONALD BROWN

BISHOP'S BREW

INGREDIENTS

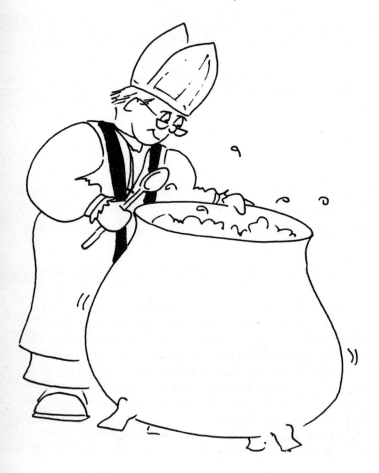

Chapter 1

GIGGLES AND GAITERS

A Bishop was visiting a primary school.

'I'll give a penny to the boy or girl who tells me who I am,' he proclaimed.

A small boy said: 'Please Sir, you are God.'

'No, I am not,' said the Bishop, 'but here's twopence.'

* * *

Country Verger to visitor admiring carved wooden bosses on altar rail: 'Don't touch them knobs. They are 'oly knobs. Last time Bishop came 'e 'adn't got 'is glasses an' 'e confirmed two o' they!'

* * *

A Bishop was annoyed one evening when his driver suggested, as they approached a church, that he should write a new sermon for his Deanery Visitations, as he had heard the current address no less than twenty-seven times. 'You preach it then, since you know it so well,' said the Bishop. The Chauffeur took up the offer enthusiastically, donning the mitre, and the Bishop exchanged his cope and staff for the driver's coat.

Sure enough, the driver delivered the oft-used homily word perfect, and with such power that the congregation

1

were obviously moved by it. New-found confidence caused the 'Bishop' to ask for 'Any Questions?' 'What,' asked a Church-warden, 'is the major thrust behind ongoing eschatalogical debate in the twentieth century?' ''Pon my word,' said the bogus Bishop, 'this parish is in dire need of a lay training programme. Even my Chauffeur, who's sitting behind you, could answer that one.'

* * *

One Bishop to another Bishop in the dole queue: 'Long time no see.'

* * *

A Vicar was expecting his Bishop for lunch after a Confirmation Service. His wife asked their daughter to lay the table for the meal before they went off to the Service. On returning, the Bishop was shown into the Dining Room where, to the Vicar's and his wife's dismay, there was no cutlery for the Bishop. On being asked the reason for this omission, the daughter replied, 'Well, I didn't think he would need cutlery as you've always said that the Bishop eats like a horse.'

* * *

A former Dean of York was the owner of a stumpy-tailed Fox Terrier, which he called Mark. When asked why his pet deserved such a name, he explained, 'The New Testament contains Life Stories of Our Lord by Matthew, Mark, Luke and John. Of the four tales, Mark's is the shortest.'

There is a story attributed to Bishop Henry Montgomery Campbell, who enjoyed a reputation as an after-dinner speaker. He had to decline an invitation to speak at a dinner because he was already booked to go somewhere else, so was asked by the dinner organiser if he could recommend a wit who could be guaranteed to make an entertaining speech. The Bishop said he didn't know a wit but he had in his Diocese several half-wits and wondered if two of them would do instead.

* * *

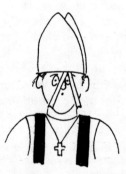

A Lancashire Bishop was rather surprised on one occasion to have his mitre suddenly whipped off by a very High Church Server for the reading of the Gospel. He was even more surprised when it was pushed back on immediately afterwards for it came from behind and sat on his head the wrong way round, with the lappets hanging over his eyes. The Server realised what he had done and started to turn it round. 'Steady on, Lad,' said the Bishop, 'it doesn't screw on, you know.'

* * *

3

If your Church roof's leakin,
Or your Hall floor's creakin,
Or your Warden's not speakin,
Or your Curate's cheekin,
Or your Bishop's no beacon,
Before you weaken,
Consult the Archdeacon.

* * *

It was Sunday morning and the Bishop of Chester was to preach at the Eucharist. In the Vestry he asked the Incumbent, 'Do you have the lavabo?' 'Yes,' he replied. So, when the moment came in the Service, the Bishop turned to the Server and said with a raise of his eyebrows 'Lavabo?' 'What?' replied the Server. 'Lavabo?' repeated the Bishop. 'What?' replied the server for the second time. 'Skip it,' said the Bishop. Later, over lunch, as the Server was the Incumbent's son, the young man enlightened the Bishop. "Mi Dad says, 'Wash mi 'ands, Lad!'."

It was fire not water that concerned the same Bishop soon afterwards.

The young Cub was committed with the task of swinging the incense. Unfortunately, his enthusiasm overtook his skill. The incense was soon on the carpet and flames were leaping up around his feet. His war-dance to put out the flames reduced his fellow Cubs in the front pew to helpless mirth. The Bishop had heard of being on fire for the Gospel but . . .!

* * *

It is said that Norfolk folk are not known for their adaptability. The present Bishop of Norwich was told the

4

only way to lead the people of his Diocese was to find out first which way they were going and then walk in front of them.

* * *

Custard Christians get upset over trifles.

* * *

Guy Warman was much loved as Bishop of Manchester, though he was something of a martinet. In one particular church, two pillars blocked the ends of the front pews on either side. When confirmation candidates came up one way and tried to get back into the pews the other way, they obviously had difficulty. The Bishop complained about this arrangement after a Confirmation Service.

The following year, the Vicar gave instructions to the Churchwardens that the two front pews should be left empty. He was annoyed and somewhat apprehensive when he processed in before the Bishop to find that as usual candidates were in the front pews on both sides. The moment arrived when the first of the newly confirmed were trying to get back into their places, some even trying to climb over the pew end. The Bishop was obviously furious. 'Do something about those pillars,' he hissed. Quick as a flash, the Vicar replied, 'Sorry, My Lord, but mi name's Wrigley not Samson!'

* * *

Bishop Luke Paget of Chester was sitting in a 'bus one day when he heard himself mentioned in a conversation that was going on between two ladies in the seat in front. 'Well, if you've never seen the Bishop of Chester you should try to have a look at him sometime, for they say he's the ugliest man in England.' The good Bishop leaned forward, tapped the lady on the shoulder and said, 'Excuse me, Madam, but anyone who says that has never seen my brother, Francis, Bishop of Oxford, for he is even worse.'

* * *

Bishop Victor Whitsey was getting more and more irritated during a Service by the antics of a very officious Server. His mitre ribbons had been straightened half-a-dozen times; his cope had been pulled this way and that; books had been thrust at him or snatched from him, and there had been a succession of flourishing bows before him. He waited for his opportunity, which came with Cardinal Newman's hymn, 'I was made a Christian when my name was given'. 'Come here, Lad,' he said, beckoning at the same time with his finger. 'Can you hear what they are singing? When I was baptised they called me Victor, but if you carry on as you are, they'll be changing that. Knock off all this fidgeting or we'll end up as Morecambe and Wise.'

* * *

From a Diocesan News Sheet: 'You will all be pleased to hear that the Bishop is making slow progress after his recent operation.'

* * *

It is not generally known that there is an angel in heaven

whose job it is to polish up the Pearly Gates and Holy Stone the celestial threshold, but it is a fact!

One day, St. Peter sent for the angel and said, 'The Bishop of Barchester is due up here tomorrow. Make sure everything is spic and span.' The angel was upset. 'We get hundreds of people up here every day,' he said, 'and they never complain. What's so special about the Bishop of Barchester?' 'Yes, I know,' said St. Peter, 'we get thousands but the arrival of a Bishop is a very rare event.'

* * *

A former Bishop of Chester's cook was complimented upon her cheerful hymn singing in the early mornings. 'I like "The Church's one Foundation" best' she said— 'One verse for soft-boiled; two verses for hard-boiled.'

* * *

A rather poverty-stricken Vicar wrote to his Bishop to complain about the cellar at the Vicarage. 'Completely flooded,' the Vicar wrote, 'and my poor hens that lived down there are all drowned.' The Bishop was very helpful. He solved the problem in two words—'Keep Ducks.'

* * *

A former Bishop of Reading tells of an occasion when he was visiting a vicarage in his area. Whilst the Vicar was out of the room, the small daughter of the house asked the Bishop, 'Can you tell me something my Daddy cannot understand?' The Bishop replied, 'Well, I will certainly try, dear.' The child continued, 'My Daddy is constantly saying to my Mummy that he cannot understand how you became a Bishop.'

* * *

One of the earliest 'funnies' concerning a Bishop must be the one contained in a letter written by the normally saintly and warm-hearted Theodoret in the year AD444. He is commenting on the death of Archbishop Cyril of Alexandria. He writes: 'At last, with a final struggle, the villain has passed way. Observing that his malice increased daily and injured the body of the Church, the Governor of our souls has lopped him off like a canker. His departure delights the survivors, but possibly disheartens the dead; there is some fear that under the provocation of his company they may send him back again to us. Care must therefore be taken to order the Guild of Undertakers to place a very big and heavy stone on his grave to stop him coming back here. I am glad and rejoice to see the fellowship of the Church delivered from such a contagion; but I am saddened and sorry as I reflect that the wretched man never took rest from his misdeeds, and died designing greater and worse.'

* * *

In recent times, a Bishop of Birkenhead visited all the Church Schools in the Diocese of Chester, accompanied by a Canon. Written accounts of these visits by children included:

'He pretended to be a Bishop but I know *real* Bishops wear big hats.'

'A bus-stop in a purple shirt came to our school and he brought a cannibal with him.'

'He came and stood there with this man and told us all about the Crook.'

* * *

Dr. Robert Runcie, Archbishop of Canterbury, tells this story about an incident when he was Bishop of St. Albans. He was on his way to an evening engagement when he happened to see some fine hams hanging in a butcher's shop in the high street of a village through which he was passing. The shop was still open and he asked his driver to hurry and buy one before the shop closed. He himself followed behind. He was just in time to hear the butcher say, 'Certainly, the Bishop can have one with pleasure; and if he can get rid of our present Vicar, I'll send him the whole d... pig.'

* * *

Another story about the Archbishop comes from the time when he was a Curate in Birmingham. He did not relish house-to-house visiting and found it rather difficult. Nevertheless, he was sent out regularly on this kind of pastoral work. He says he would often ring a door-bell and then pray that nobody would answer for he never knew what to say.

* * *

A former Bishop of Gloucester had a defective memory and on one celebrated occasion was walking round a

9

Garden Party at his home greeting the clergy. 'My dear fellow,' he said to one clergyman, 'how lovely to see you here today; and how is your dear wife?' The clergyman, rather surprised, replied, 'She's dead, my Lord. Don't you remember, you wrote me a very helpful letter at the time?' 'I am so sorry,' the Bishop exclaimed, 'do, please, forgive me.' He moved on. Later that afternoon the Bishop came across the same man again. 'Hello,' he exclaimed, 'good to have you with us and how is your dear wife?' 'Still dead, my Lord,' said the priest, 'still dead.'

* * *

The Bishop had preached at Harvest Festival and as he stood at the door, people were very complimentary about his sermon. 'Splendid,' said one: 'Thank you for the wonderful message,' said another, and so it went on. However, one rather shabbily dressed man took the Bishop's hand and said, 'Pathetic,' before moving out. The compliments started again, but after a few minutes the strange man was back in the queue. This time he said to the Bishop, 'Very, very boring,' and again went through the door. The pattern repeated itself yet again. This time the message was, 'Hope it will be a long time before we see you again.' Soon everyone had gone except the Churchwarden. 'Who was that strange man?' asked the Bishop. 'He said some very peculiar things.' 'Don't worry about him,' came the reply, 'he's a bit simple and he just wanders round repeating what he hears other people say.'

* * *

At a special Thanksgiving Service at St. Stephen's, Flowery Field, for the completion of the remodelled church, the Vicar invited the congregation to turn round and face the plaque at the back, using the familiar northern shortened 'a'. Bishop Whitsey commented publicly with: "I am glad, Vicar, you said 'the plaque at the back' (short 'a's) and not the 'plaaque at the baack'. It sounds much better."

* * *

Report from Synod: A shiver went round the Bench of Bishops, trying to find a spine to run down!

* * *

Almost a century ago, there was a rather daunting Archbishop of Canterbury: valiant for the truth; terrifying to the false, the work-shy and the pretentious; he was also rather difficult to entertain and the clergy were none too keen on the privilege! On one occasion, the honour fell upon a certain Vicar and his wife, who were determined to do it well. They spent anxious days preparing the menu and the bedchamber. They believed their efforts had succeeded, for when His Grace made his farewells, he thanked them most warmly for their kindness. The Vicar's wife was emboldened to say that she hoped he would do them the honour again sometime, 'And you must bring your wife too, for she would be most welcome.' Host and hostess were somewhat discomfited when the Archbishop answered in his honest and uncompromising way: 'No Ma'am, no. I don't mind roughing it meself; but I cannot ask mi wife to do so too.'

* * *

Episcopal subtleties to persuade another bishop to take into his Diocese a priest who is not altogether satisfactory, are not unknown. This is a practice known in the trade as 'Throwing dead cats over the garden-fence'. For instance, one bone-idle Curate is commended in this way—'And the Vicar who gets this young man to work with him will be extremely fortunate'.

The priest who is too mean to give anyone even a cup of tea gets a push with 'A man of rare gifts'.

The crackpot priest is described as 'well-balanced' and the Bishop answers the quizzical look of his Secretary with, 'Well, he has chips on *both* shoulders!'

* * *

When William Temple was Bishop of Manchester he received a letter several days late. It had been redirected several times. It was addressed to 'William Temple, The Palace, Manchester'. The address had been crossed out and replaced with 'Not known at The Palace, try The Opera House'. He also said that during his time in Manchester he received a bill from the Laundry for washing one of his surplices. This had been described as 'To washing one Bell Tent—2/6d'.

* * *

Definition: Suffragan Bishop—'A second fiddle in a one-man band'.

* * *

A Bishop of London was seated next to the French

Ambassador when a fly settled on the tablecloth. Although the conversation had been in English, the Bishop was keen to show off his knowledge of French. 'Le mouche,' he said, airily. After a brief glance, the Ambassador said, '*La* mouche'. The Bishop looked hard at the insect from this and that angle. Finally he exclaimed, 'I must say you've got remarkably good eyesight!'

* * *

Nathanial: 'Daddy, how do you become a Bishop?'
(aged 7)

Daddy: 'Well, no-one seems to actually know, but a good first step is to be ordained. Do you want to be a Vicar when you grow up?'

Nathanial: 'Well, not really—only if I have to to be a Bishop.'

* * *

Overheard:

"On January 21st, the Bishop will speak on 'Twelve Cheers for the Church of England'."
"Lor'," said one Liverpudlian, "I 'ope they'll be more comfortable than these 'ard wooden pews!"

* * *

Bishop's letter to retiring priest:

'And finally, I have pleasure in making you Canon

13

Emeritus.' An aside to his Secretary: 'And I do hope he knows what "Emeritus" means—"e" means "gone", "finished": and "meritus" means "deservedly so".'

* * *

The sudden illness of an incumbent necessitated a telegram to the Bishop. In the emergency, the Bishop came and took the Service himself. Afterwards, two very much over-awed Churchwardens felt that they must express their thanks to the Bishop. This they did in the following words: 'My Lord, we greatly appreciate your great kindness in coming to us; a poorer preacher would have done, but we couldn't find one.'

* * *

A Cathedral Canon used to hold family prayers in his home. After duly praying for the Bishop of the Diocese, for the Dean and for his fellow Canons, he would say, 'And now we pray for the Minor Canons of this Cathedral Church, for they also are Thy creatures.'

* * *

When Geoffrey Fisher was Bishop of Chester, he arrived at Bishop's House one day in 1939 after a meeting on the Wirral to be told by his Secretary that twenty evacuees had been sent to the house for board and lodging. This explained the very loud noise that was emanating from upstairs. The Bishop was obviously annoyed that they were creating such a disturbance. He pounded up the stairs, two at a time, flung open the door and roared,

"QUIET!" No-one took a bit of notice and the noise continued unabated. It is said that this was a very important lesson for the Bishop. He discovered at that moment that 'the world' did not respond to his strictures as readily as the boys at Repton School.

* * *

A Victorian Archbishop, taking his last Confirmation, said, 'I declare this stone well and truly laid.' (Authority—his successor).

* * *

Bishop Henry Montgomery Campbell of London used to say he hated meetings of all kinds. 'Waste of time,' he would snort. On one occasion, he went into a Board of Finance Meeting intoning: 'We brought nothing into this Meeting and it is certain we can carry nothing out.' But then he brightened up a bit—'Must admit I've had a good day today,' he said. 'Really enjoyed it—I've been out in the Diocese to bury a Vicar.'

* * *

Archbishop Trench of Dublin retired at a great age. His successor invited him to dinner. Because the old man was not adaptable to change, he and his wife were placed at the head and foot of the table, the places to which they had been accustomed. At the end of the meal, still obviously thinking himself in his own house, the old gentleman observed to his wife, 'My dear, I fear that this cook cannot be counted among our successes.'

A Bishop of Kimberley and Kuruman, who had a well-developed sense of humour, was leaving the Diocese. A farewell was held in the Town Hall. The chairman of this gathering said that he was sorry that some who had hoped to be present had not been able to come. He quoted the line of an evening hymn, 'Some are sick and some are sad'. The Bishop, in a whisper to a friend on the platform, said: "He may as well continue, 'And some have never loved thee well. And some have lost the love they had'."

* * *

A lady sitting next to a Bishop at dinner observed in the course of conversation, 'My aunt was prevented at the last moment from sailing in the ship which foundered here last week. Would you not call that the intervention of providence?' 'I cannot tell,' replied the Bishop, 'for I do not know your aunt.'

* * *

Why are Archdeacons always on the move?
Because they know that if they stopped someone would hit them!

* * *

Bishop Eric Tracey, while still Bishop of Wakefield, was due to go into hospital. A woman, who was attending a Diocesan Meeting, expressed concern for the Bishop and hoped it was 'nothing very serious'. He tried to reassure her: 'O, no, it's nothing very much,' he said, 'just haemorrhoids, actually.' 'You poor man,' replied the woman, 'all the speaking you have to do and having a sore throat all the time.' The Bishop smiled gently, but later confessed to a friend, 'You know she might be right. Medical science is so advanced these days that they may well tackle the problem from that end!'

* * *

When Walter Frere was Bishop of Truro, a Vicar invited him to stay the night after a Confirmation. Before supper, Frere was walking down a dimly-lit passage in the Vicarage when the Vicar's wife, coming up from behind, gave him a clout over the ear, with the remark: 'That'll teach you to ask the Bishop to stay when we've nothing in the house.'

* * *

When William Greer was retiring from the See of Manchester, he said that although he would miss many things, there was one aspect of his life which would be improved by his laying down the burden of office. 'For years,' he confessed, 'I have found it embarrassing to sign an hotel register with the names 'William Manchester' and 'Marigold Greer.'

* * *

The Bishop was the dinner guest. The table beautifully prepared and the food looked delicious. They were ready to begin. The hostess spoke to her daughter, aged six. 'Mary, you say Grace, please.' A rather long delay ensued. The mother coaxed the little girl, 'Come on,

Mary, say what you heard me say this morning at breakfast.' In a loud voice it came out, 'O God, why did I invite the Bishop to dinner tonight?'

* * *

Lucius, sometime Bishop of Knaresborough, was usually known (privately) as Luscious. When, as Vicar of Macclesfield, he was to be promoted to the episcopate, he went round to explain and say goodbye to parishioners. A dear old lady said, 'Oh, Vicar, it is we old women who will miss you most. We always feel that you are one of us.'
Another parishioner, as the future Bishop announced his threefold promotion—Canon-Residentiary of Ripon, Archdeacon of Richmond, Bishop of Knaresborough—commented tartly, 'That's pleurisy, ain't it?'

* * *

A Bishop of Carlisle was terminating an interview with a very difficult woman of the diocese who was at Rose Castle once again to lodge a complaint about something or other. They were in the hall, getting round to the final handshake, when a Secretary went out slamming the door. The Bishop's wife called downstairs: 'Has that stupid woman finally gone, dear?' Quick as a flash, the Bishop replied, 'O, yes, my love, she went ages ago. I'm with Mrs. Robinson now.'

* * *

Chester Cathedral choirboy sitting down to tea and being questioned by his mother about Evensong, from which he had just returned.

'Who was the Preacher?' she enquired.
'The Bishop of Birkenhead.'
'What did he preach about?'
'Don't know. He didn't tell us.'

*   *   *

A one-time Bishop of Birmingham once preached a sermon, which was well-publicised, in which he described certain practices of the Roman Catholic Church as 'magic'. A few nights later, he went out at a late hour to post some letters and, in the darkness, espied a cleric on the opposite side of the road, whom he thought he recognised. On being hailed by the Bishop, the figure crossed over towards him and said, 'I am sorry, my Lord, but you are mistaken. I am not of your flock. I am the local magician!'

*   *   *

A Welsh Priest writes:

I remember Bishop Victor Whitsey asking me to attend a Meeting. It was on a Saturday afternoon about six weeks away and I remember saying to him, 'I am terribly sorry, my Lord, I cannot go, I have a funeral.' He said, 'A funeral! What do you mean? It's six weeks away.' 'I know,' I said, 'I am hoping to bury fifteen Englishmen at Twickenham.'

*   *   *

After the death of Prince Albert, while the Queen was in

deep sorrow, there was a Bishop at Windsor who tried to comfort her. 'Do remember, ma'am,' he said, 'that Jesus Christ is now your husband.' The Queen paused for a moment before replying: 'That, Bishop, is TWADDLE, ABSOLUTE TWADDLE!'

* * *

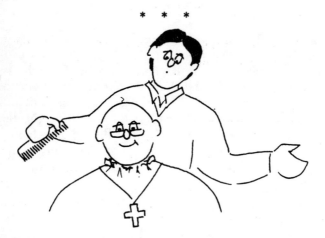

A Bishop, who shall be nameless, with three hairs on his head, went to the barber:

'I want a shampoo and blow-dry, please.'
'Very good, sir.'
Afterwards—'On which side shall I part it, sir?'
'On the left, please.'
After a moment's consternation—'I'm very sorry, sir, but one of your hairs has come out.'
'Oh, that's all right. Part it in the middle.'
After another moment of anguish: 'I'm frightfully sorry, sir, but another one has come out.'
'Don't worry,' said the Bishop, 'just leave it rough!'

* * *

A Bishop of Manchester once gave his bachelor curates some advice about finding the right kind of wife. He said, 'Find a woman who is pretty, prudent and with private means, and make sure these are in reverse order of importance!'

* * *

A Suffragan Bishop is not so much deprived of a Cathedral as relieved of a Dean.

* * *

Bishop Hensley Henson of Durham emerged from a meeting of clergy wives at the Town Hall in Sunderland. He stood on the top step outside the building, raised his head to heaven and in a loud voice called out, 'You were wrong, Paul, it is better to burn!' (Reference: 1 Corinthians, VII, 9).

* * *

When Bishop Paget was getting ready to retire, he entertained Geoffrey Fisher, his successor-elect, who had come to look round the house. Fisher stood with hands together and eyes closed waiting for Grace before lunch. 'Sit down, Geoffrey,' said Paget, 'and get on with it. We only say Grace in this house for potatoes.'

* * *

When Geoffrey Fisher first arrived in the Chester Diocese as its Bishop, he went to several House Parties, which had

21

been arranged in stately homes, so that he could meet people who might be encouraged to give money towards an appeal he had made for new churches. It is said that at one of these he came down very early to breakfast; the only other person at the table was a little girl. He charged his plate at the sideboard and sat next to her. To break the silence, he asked her to name the Sacraments. As soon as she had answered, he asked her about Holy Orders and the number and types of Ministers in the Church. When she had answered, he went back to the sideboard, collected some toast for the little girl and another cup of coffee for himself, and asked her to repeat the Apostles' Creed. When this had been completed, he asked for the Nicene Creed. 'Mmm,' he said, 'you are a clever little girl, so I am going to ask you one more question: can you repeat the Athanasian Creed?' Elizabeth-Anne looked his Lordship in the eye: 'Dammit,' she said, 'do remember I am only seven!'

* * *

'Let us drink the Loyal Toast—I give you, "The queer old dean"!'—Canon Spooner.

* * *

Archbishop Geoffrey Fisher used to enjoy telling two stories concerning the Press. The first was about a visit to the United States aboard the Queen Elizabeth. As soon as the ship docked, a swarm of reporters arrived to interview him. He prided himself on his ability to parry awkward questions. Within seconds, one was flung at him: 'Archbishop, do you intend to visit the Night Clubs in New York?' With a wry smile, the Archbishop countered with, 'Why, are there any Night Clubs in New York?' His self-congratulation lasted until the morning papers arrived. A banner headline said, 'ARCHBISHOP WANTS TO KNOW'. The report began, 'The very first question the Archbishop of Canterbury asked on his arrival yesterday was, 'Are there any Night Clubs in New York?'

It was a British Daily that figured in another story. For some time it had expressed its disapproval of the Archbishop. One day it carried a headline 'The Archbishop must go!' A week later, the paper was incensed again by a speech he had made. Another headline—this time it said, 'The Archbishop has gone too far.'

* * *

In one of his pastoral letters, Bishop Victor Whitsey said he expected the clergy to wear clerical collars when they were on duty in parish and diocese. When the Bishop retired, the wags of the Diocese said that although they were sorry to see him go, they were relieved that the accident rate on the Runcorn Bridge would be diminished, for clergy would no longer have to take their hands off the wheel to put on a clerical collar as they came into Chester for an episcopal interview.

* * *

Bishop Richard Hanson, fine scholar that he was, became convinced that he had solved one of the great mysteries connected with the Church of England. The question that no one had been able to answer was: 'Why does everyone in the Anglican Church want to sit in the back pews?' The Bishop said he was convinced that it all went back to our

23

ancestors, the cavemen. They cowered at the back of their caves while horrors appeared at the front!

* * *

The Bishop of Barking was once on a platform with a group of other people at a School Speech Day. The lady presenting the prizes rose to perform her part in the event, but as she came forward she tripped over a loose floorboard and fell. The Bishop was just able to catch her before she hit the floor. 'Well, well,' he said, 'this is the first time I have ever had a fallen woman in my arms.' She was just as quick: 'This is a first for me too,' she said, 'for I've never been picked up by a Bishop before.'

* * *

The Bishop looked down from the platform at the large number of clergy present for a special meeting. He said to the Dean, 'This looks a very scriptural gathering.' 'Do you mean they all look like keen disciples?' 'Oh no,' said the Bishop, 'I suspect we have here the multitude that loafs and fishes.'

* * *

Chapter 2

VICARS, CURATES AND OTHER GREEN THINGS UPON THE EARTH

It is alleged that in the 1800s the people of Wallasey made a living from wrecking. One Sunday night, rockets were heard. The Vicar interrupted his sermon and shouted, 'Warden, lock the door. I must have time to get my robes off. We must all start equal.'

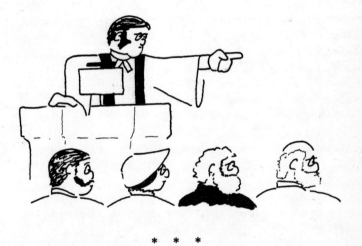

* * *

A Curate was delighted to discover that 'pepsi-cola' is an anagram of episcopal. He wrote and told the Bishop of his discovery, stressing that 'sparkle and refreshment' seemed to make it so very appropriate. His Vicar agreed that it was most appropriate but said this was because it was 'full of gas and lacking in taste'.

* * *

Jonathan, being the youngest son at the Vicarage, then aged 7, was somewhat concerned when Mummy went back to paid employment after several years at home. After three days of this new experience, he came into the bedroom at 7.30 a.m. to find Mummy getting ready for work and Dad still lying in bed. When asked if he was getting used to the idea of Mummy going to work, he replied: 'Yes, it's O.K. but what will we do if Daddy ever gets a job?'

* * *

Confidences beget Confidences:

'For years,' confessed the Deacon, 'I thought Dan and Beersheba were husband and wife.'

'Don't worry,' confessed the Curate. 'For years I thought the Epistles were the brothers of the Apostles!'

The Vicar said nothing. For years he had imagined the Sermon on the Mount to be instructions to a jockey before 'the off'!

* * *

As he made his way down the street, the Vicar was smiling to himself. 'You seem very contented with life, Vicar,' said a parishioner who met him. 'I am,' was the reply, 'and so would you be in my case. I have made seven hearts happy today.' 'How was that?' 'Why, I've just married three couples.' 'But that only accounts for six.' 'Well, you don't think I did it for nothing, do you?'

* * *

One Saturday evening in 1987, an incumbent in Macclesfield gave a parishioner a lift to the railway station. The only place he could stop was alongside the taxi rank. The passenger got out and thanked the Vicar. He was about to drive off when suddenly the rear door was opened and another lady got in. 'Take me to the Stanley Hotel quickly, please,' she said. Without a word, the Vicar drove the five miles to the requested destination. The lady got out and came to the car window. 'I am not a taxi driver, madam. In fact, I am the Vicar.' 'Oh,' she said, and hastily pushed back into her purse the five-pound note she had extracted. Instead, she produced a fifty pence piece. 'Put that in the collection tomorrow from me,' she said. The Vicar thanked her and started to drive off. She ran alongside, tapping at the window. Again he wound it down. 'You couldn't come for me just after midnight and take me back to the station, could you?'

* * *

John, the Curate, announced that he was moving on from the church, and a few days later the Vicar was stopped in the public library by a worried-looking parishioner. 'Is it true that John is leaving?' she asked. 'I'm afraid so,' replied the Vicar. 'Oh, I am sorry. 'E does a lovely funeral and I wanted him to do mine. 'E gets 'em all crying and I want 'em all to cry at my funeral.'

27

Diocesan Secretary to plaintive incumbent:
'What do you mean, in lieu of a stipend increase you would prefer Sundays off?'

* * *

The strangest man in the parish was the old Colonel who lived near the church. He confessed to the Vicar that he thought the reason for his longevity was that every morning he sprinkled gunpowder on his cornflakes instead of sugar. He was well in his nineties when he died. He left a widow and three sons; and a very large crater where the crematorium used to stand.

* * *

A Vicar looked at his diary and read, '9.30 a.m. H.C.' So, he went to church, put on his robes and got ready for the service. Not a single person arrived. He couldn't understand it until he got home and his wife said, 'I thought you were having your hair cut this morning.'

* * *

First Man: 'Our Vicar has got foot and mouth disease.'

Second Man: 'I didn't know humans could get that.'

First Man: 'Well, he's got it—can't preach and won't visit.'

* * *

'George,' said a country Vicar to one of his parishioners, 'why is it that immediately after Evensong you go straight across the road and into the "King's Head"?' 'Well, Vicar,' said George, 'I suppose it's what you would call a "thirst after righteousness".'

* * *

In the grim days of 1939 and 1940, notices about National Service were posted up in Employment Exchanges throughout Great Britain. The official message stated that 'All persons in the above age-groups are required to register for national service except lunatics, the blind and Ministers of Religion.' Some felt it was a very appropriate grouping!

* * *

A very difficult man in the parish had a row with the Vicar. In spite of the provocation, the Vicar controlled his temper and again and again answered him mildly. This seemed to make the man even more angry and he finally produced his last insult. 'If I had an imbecile son,' he said, 'I would send him into the Church as a clergyman.' The Vicar quickly replied with: 'I can only say how pleased I am that your father did not have the same view.'

* * *

The Vicar took his little daughter with him visiting one day. Granny Smith made them very welcome. She was asked by the little girl how old she was. 'Do you know,

dear,' the old lady said, 'I can't remember my age.'
'Well,' said the little girl, 'if I were you I would look in
your knickers for it says in mine "For three and four-year
olds".'

* * *

Some months ago, a Curate was giving his four-year-old
daughter a cuddle before she went to bed. As he picked
her up and squeezed her tight, she said, 'Daddy, you're so
strong! I really think you'll be God one day!'

* * *

A Cheshire Vicar had two cats. Their names were Ancient
and Modern. The Vicar said this was because they were
both hims.

* * *

A South African priest, now working in England, tells
how he once attended a Rural Deanery Lunch there. A
cold buffet was the order of the day. Standing eating the
cold chicken, he asked the Archdeacon, 'Have you seen
the colour of your chicken?' It was a distinct shade of
liturgical green. The Archdeacon looked in horror and
then glanced at the questioner's plate. Both discovered
with horror that they were consuming green chicken and
decided the best plan of action was to feed the chicken to
the dog that was languishing in the African sun just off
the verandah. They then glanced around and everyone
else's chicken appeared green, and chortled to themselves.
'We will be all right this afternoon; heaven help the

others.' It was only while eating Vanilla Ice Cream, which also appeared green, that they realised they were standing under green plastic sheeting over the verandah which, because of the sunlight, made everything appear slightly tinted (green). There was much laughter, but it was generally agreed that the dog 'had the last laugh' as he readily enjoyed the 'green chicken'.

* * *

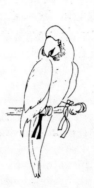

The Vicar was visiting a new parishioner when he noticed her parrot. It had a red ribbon tied around one leg, and a blue ribbon round the other. 'I like your parrot,' said the Vicar, 'but what are the ribbons for?' 'They are to do with my faith, Vicar,' replied Miss Pringle. 'How do you mean?' asked the cleric. 'Well, when my faith feels strong, I pull the red ribbon, and the parrot sings "Onward Christian Soldiers"; and when my faith is weak, I pull the blue ribbon and the parrot sings "Abide with me".' 'Interesting,' said the Vicar. 'What happens when you pull both ribbons?' This time the parrot replied: 'I fall off the perch, you idiot.'

* * *

The B.B.C. issued a storm warning and because of the wide-spread storms advised anyone who had to go out to wear something white so that they would be clearly seen by motorists. The Vicar had to go to visit a sick parishioner. He put his surplice over his raincoat. Alas, he was knocked down by a snow plough!

*   *   *

Mummy had heard dear little Montmorency utter a swear word and that was too, too awful because Daddy was the Vicar. 'Off you go straight to bed, you naughty, naughty boy,' she said. 'No tea for you, and just wait until Daddy hears about this!' When Daddy arrived home, Mummy told him the sorry tale. 'He swore, did he?' said Daddy. 'I'll teach him to swear,' and he set off up the stairs. Unfortunately, Montmorency had left one of his roller skates on the next-to-the-top step and Daddy came crashing down again. After almost five minutes of invective, during which Daddy never repeated himself once, Mummy said, 'All right, Daddy, that will do for the first lesson.'

*   *   *

A Vicar, giving out the notices, said, 'The Collections next Sunday will be for the Assistant Curate's Fund and I appeal for generous support for that object.'

*   *   *

The doctor and the parson were standing with the wife beside a dying old man's bed.

'I'm afraid he's gone,' said the priest.
'Yes, he has,' said the doctor.
'No, I baint,' murmured the patient, feebly sitting up.
'Lie down, dear,' said the wife, 'doctor and parson do know best.'

* * *

The Vicar said to the congregation on Sunday, 'You will all like to know what your contributions to the Organ Fund have bought . . .' (fishes in his pocket and pulls out a mouth organ).

* * *

'I have nothing but praise for the new Vicar.'
'I noticed that when I came round with the plate last Sunday.'

* * *

The Vicar was visiting one of his lady parishioners and rang the front door bell of her house. Despite hearing one or two noises inside the house, nobody answered the door. Before he left, he wrote on a scrap of paper, REVELA-TION, CHAPTER THREE, VERSE TWENTY ('Behold I stand at the door and knock; if anyone hears my voice and answers the door, I will come in . . .').

The following Sunday, as the lady was leaving church after the morning service, she put into the Vicar's hand a piece of paper, which had written on it: GENESIS, CHAPTER THREE, VERSE TEN ('I heard the sound of thee in the garden, and I was afraid, because I was naked; and I hid myself'). He concluded that evidently the lady was having a bath at the time!

* * *

A Curate was sternly enjoined by his Rector never again to use the expression 'The Holy Spirit' but only and always 'The Holy Ghost'. This lecture occurred at a Monday morning 'Chapter' which soon afterwards terminated as follows:

Rector: The Lord be with you.
Curate: And with thy Ghost.

* * *

A raw Curate visited a man concerning the funeral of his mother and the man asked him which Church he was from. The Curate replied: 'The Church of England.' The man's response was, 'Church of England? Isn't that a bit like the Christian Church?'

* * *

A phone call came to the Cricket Club asking urgently for the Vicar, who was a keen player. The phone in the pavilion was answered by a member. 'Hold the line,' he said. 'Hold the line. The Vicar's just gone in to bat. He'll be back in a minute.'

* * *

Our Vicar left three months ago so we gave him a little momentum from the parish.

*　*　*

The Vicar was busily showing visitors around his rather ornate church, where major repairs were being carried out to the roofing timbers. As he pointed out the decorative wooden statues and flying-angels surrounding the ceiling, a workman, high on the scaffolding, accidentally hit his thumb with a hammer. This painful occurrence provoked a stream of language which was, to say the least, 'colourful', and clearly heard by everybody below. The Vicar (who happened to be an amateur ventriloquist) felt a rebuke was not only called for but should be of such a nature as to make a lasting impression upon the culprit. 'Throwing' his voice upwards, he made a gilded, female flying-angel seem to say: 'Now, now, my man, that's not the kind of language to use in the House of God.' The astonished carpenter could scarcely believe his ears, and calling to the Foreman said, 'Did you hear that, Boss?—it was only ten minutes ago I drove a six-inch nail into her backside and she didn't say a word.'

*　*　*

George Ingle, Bishop of Willesden, made this remark when he was speaking at a Clergy Meeting in Edgware. 'No-one is infallible—not even the youngest Curate present!'

*　*　*

There was once a poor curate who was bemoaning his impecunious state in the hearing of his Vicar. 'Never mind,' came the rejoinder, 'the fringe benefits are out of this world.'

* * *

While knocking at the door of an elderly gentleman's flat in his parish, the Vicar saw a little girl running into the next flat and heard her say to her grandmother that there was a man knocking at Mr. X's door. The Vicar got no reply and the grandmother came out to tell him that the old gentleman was out. He thanked her and as he turned to leave he overheard her say to her granddaughter, 'That's not a man; it's a clergyman.'

* * *

The Vicar's small daughter was seen burying a dead bird in the garden: 'In the Name of the Father, and of the Son, and into the hole he goes. Amen.'

* * *

The Vicar was known to be a scholar. The reason was that it was difficult to understand his sermons! At the Harvest Festival, the Vicar felt that even this occasion should not pass by without the congregation being reminded of his learning and wisdom. After expressing his personal views on a difficult theological question, he concluded: 'I am afraid that commentators disagree with me.' The next day, the Vicar found a sack at his door, together with the following note: 'I understand 'common taters' don't agree with you so I am letting you have this sack of King Edwards.'

* * *

The housewife opens the door to the Vicar. She is in her housecoat and behind her is all the debris left by three just-vanished schoolchildren. 'O, my God!' she says in horror. 'Afraid not,' comes the reply, 'He doesn't do house calls so He sent me instead.'

* * *

Two clergymen talking together:

'My congregation took a collection for my Continuing Ministerial Education. Do you know of any Conference for £2.26?'

* * *

Shortly before leaving his parish, two small boys stopped the Vicar and said:

'You're leaving, Vicar, aren't you?'
'That's right.'
'Are you leaving tomorrow?'
'Don't be silly, Jimmy,' his friend nudged him.
'No, there's a few weeks yet,' said the Vicar.
'And then will they pull the church down?'

* * *

Chain letters are usually regarded as highly undesirable, but maybe church-goers would make an exception in the case of this one:

First Church's Name: . . . .

Second Church's Name: . . . .

Are you dissatisfied with your Vicar? If so, parcel him up and send him to the first Church named above. Then write 130 copies of this letter and send them to any churches of your choice, deleting the first church's name and adding that of your own church. Eventually, you will receive 16,900 vicars—one of them *should* suit you! Be warned—do *not* break the chain or you may get your own Vicar back again.

* * *

The Funeral Director's car was waiting outside the Chapel after the Service and, having made arrangements to be transported, the Vicar sat himself in the front passenger seat. Because of the head rest, he was not readily visible from the rear of the vehicle. Having loaded the flowers into the Estate Wagon through the back door, the rather impatient driver posed the question, 'Now where's the b...y Vicar?' and got the shock of his life when a voice from the front seat replied, 'The b...y Vicar's here.'

* * *

A wife awakening her husband said 'It is time to get up!' 'Why?' he asked. She replied: 'Firstly, it is 8.30 a.m. Secondly, it is Sunday, and thirdly, you are the Vicar.'

A golf-crazy Vicar, after browbeating his congregation about keeping the Lord's Day holy, sneaks off to his local golf course on a Sunday afternoon, knowing that his flock will not be there. But heaven is not to be fooled in such matters and the angel Gabriel, on spotting him, storms into the Almighty's presence, demanding retribution for such hypocrisy. 'I have a plan,' says the Almighty, and promptly allows the Vicar to land a hole in one—over 400 yards. 'You can't do that,' says Gabriel. 'Just watch me,' says the Almighty, as he coaxes the next shot out of a bunker, across a green, between two trees and straight into the hole. Gabriel can see the Vicar going into ecstasy on the golf course and is furious with God. 'You should be punishing him,' he screams, 'not helping him!' 'Ah, but I am punishing him,' says the Almighty. 'How's that?' says Gabriel. 'You've just given him the round of his life.' 'Ah, yes,' says the Almighty, 'but whom can he tell?'

* * *

A Yorkshire Vicar took his family to the seaside for the day. Returning home late at night, he ran out of petrol just before reaching home. Fortunately, there was a garage not far away and he knew the proprietor. When he got there, however, there was no suitable receptacle for the petrol. He returned to the car and took the only available container—the baby's potty. A few minutes later he was gingerly pouring the petrol from the potty into the tank when one of his parishioners walked by. Seeing this strange sight, the parishioner said, 'By gum, Vicar, I wish I had your faith.'

* * *

Two skeletons met in the churchyard one night. One

skeleton said, 'How are you? How long have you been dead?' 'I'm not dead,' said the second skeleton, 'I'm the Vicar.'

* * *

When there's no-one in when you call, just leave your calling card with the nicely ambiguous message—'The Vicar called and found you out!'

* * *

From the North-East comes this story:

The Vicar and the Pollis (police):

The Vicar is on his bike and the pollis puts up his hand to stop him. Squeal of brakes and the Vicar just manages to pull up in time. 'Nearly got you that time,' says Pollis. 'You'll never get me, Constable; you see God is with me. God is always with me.' 'Ah, that's it. Got you this time, Vicar,' says the pollis—'two on a bike.'

* * *

'I don't wear my collar more than absolutely necessary now in case I'm taken for an Atheist'. Episcopal clergyman.

* * *

A man was telling some hens to 'begger off . . .' The Vicar came along. 'Now, my man, you shouldn't say that . . . just say "shoo, shoo" and they'll begger off themselves.'

* * *

The Vicar had been in hospital for several weeks undergoing routine surgery and at last he was able to ask his churchwardens to let his parishioners know he was on the road to recovery. The next day people were startled to find the following announcement on the Church Notice Board: 'God is good. The Vicar is better.'

* * *

One morning, while sitting in the front pew deep in thought and meditation, a Cheshire Vicar heard a noise by the west door of his church. Had one of his flock decided to join him in the daily office? He didn't turn around but just tried to gather together the threads of the disturbed prayer thoughts. When he had eventually finished his devotions, he got up, turned around to leave and to his surprise there was no-one there. As he approached the door, he saw the reason for the noise. An envelope had been forced beneath the great door. It was addressed to 'The Occupier, St. John's Church'. The Vicar hesitated and glanced heavenward. Should he open another's mail?

41

He ventured to do so and read, 'There is no record of a T.V. Licence for your residence.' Back in his study, the Vicar appended the reply: 'The occupier has not yet installed a set. He is still using me to communicate.' That ended the correspondence.

* * *

Visitor to old church verger:

'Has the Reverend J. S. Hemmingford been here long?' 'Oh, yes,' replied the verger, 'Mr. Hemmingford has been the Incumberance here for nigh on twenty years.'

* * *

Clerical retirement doesn't reduce us all to Cleriatrics!

* * *

The Vicar of a small village received an invitation to dine one evening with the Squire. As the village was sparsely lighted, his Reverence took a lantern to light him through the dark lanes. He had a very enjoyable time and returned home safe and sound. Next morning, he received a note from the Squire: 'Dear Vicar, if you will kindly return the parrot in its cage, you can have your lantern.'

* * *

The doctor went to see her, but the Vicar didn't go:
But the doctor had been sent for, and the Vicar didn't know.

The doctor got rewarded with a handsome little cheque,
But the Vicar for not knowing simply got it in the neck.

* * *

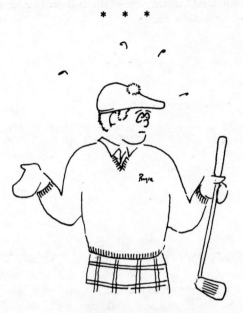

A clergyman was playing golf with a friend whose language left something to be desired. 'Damn it! Missed!' he kept saying after every air-shot as divots flew in all directions. Eventually, the clergyman felt constrained to admonish his friend. 'You know,' he said, 'if you go on like that you'll be struck down by a bolt from heaven.' All to no avail. At the next hole, the bloke took another almighty swipe at the ball and then let fly verbally as well. At once there was a flash of lightning and the clergyman disappeared in a puff of smoke. From somewhere in the clouds a voice could be heard rumbling, 'Damn it! Missed!'

* * *

From a school essay:

'... and when the marauders landed on the coast, the villagers would run to the top of the hill and set fire to the deacon ...'

*   *   *

A priest was transferred to a diocese whose bishop was renowned for being a very strict disciplinarian. His parish priest greeted him with the words: 'Welcome to the Cruel See ...'

*   *   *

There was an old clergyman so besotted with cricket that he occasionally said 'Over' instead of 'Amen'. On one celebrated occasion he walked from the lectern having proclaimed, 'Here endeth the second innings'. When he had a parish-hall built, he had signs for the doors, one of which said 'Out', the other 'Not out'. He even liked to preach on the game and his favourite texts were:

Peter stood up with the eleven and was bold.
(Acts 2–14).

I caught you by guile. (2 Cor. 12. 16).

... drinking in the pavilions. (I Kings 20. 12).

*   *   *

One of the Curate's children, the day after Daddy's XI

beat the Vicar's XI, was heard to say to his friend:
'I'll be the good batsman, you be the wicked keeper.'

* * *

Loyal wife to callers who wanted the golf-playing Vicar:
'I am sorry, the Vicar is away on a course.'

* * *

The old retired Canon had given the parish good service
during the long vacancy, but now a new Vicar was to be
instituted and there came the time for the old man's
farewell address. It was an Urban Priority Area, with
much deprivation and vandalism. Many of the church
windows were broken and had been covered over with
hardboard. It was this that was used as an illustration in
the sermon. 'These pieces of hardboard are only a substitute for panes of glass, just as I have only been a substitute
for a proper parish priest, but now, thank God, the real
thing will soon be here.' He shook hands with the
congregation as they left. One old dear tried to express
her thanks. 'Canon,' she said, 'we have never thought of
you as a substitute; we have always found you to be a real
pane.'

* * *

It was the Christmas season and the Vicar decided to ask
the children what difference it would make if Christ had
not been born. There were the expected answers—no
Christmas tree, no presents, no nativity play and so on.
After the Service, one ten-year-old boy sidled up to the

45

Vicar and said, 'If Jesus hadn't been born, you'd be out of a job.' The Vicar was glad that that point hadn't been made *during* the Service.

* * *

The Vicar announced one Sunday that he was leaving the parish to take up another post elsewhere in the Diocese. He was quite touched afterwards to find the old Verger sitting at the back of the church with head in hands and eyes full of tears. He tried to reassure him. 'Don't get upset,' he said, 'there will soon be another Vicar here and I've no doubt he will be a lot better than me.' 'Oh no, he won't,' said the old man, 'last Vicar said that when he left and it wasn't true.'

* * *

The parishioners realised they had a very good Vicar, one of the best in the Diocese. There was just one thing that puzzled them. Every Thursday they saw him walk to the Railway Station just before one o'clock and sit on the platform for a few minutes until the London express had gone through. Then he would get up and make a start on his afternoon visiting. This routine went on for a year or two before one of the Wardens asked for an explanation. 'Oh, it's quite simple,' said the Vicar. 'It does me good to watch the express train go through the station for that's the only thing that moves in this parish without my pushing it.'

* * *

'Last absolution before the M6'—Enterprising Vicar's Notice Board.

* * *

Behind every successful man there stands an astonished mother-in-law.

* * *

My friend, the Undertaker, the last person on earth to let me down.

* * *

Chapter 3

HATCHES, MATCHES AND DISPATCHES

The story is told of a bride-to-be who was extremely nervous about her wedding.day and who went to see the Vicar in order to find some reassurance. He sought to calm her fears by telling her there were only three things she needed to remember. 'Firstly,' he said, 'you need to remember the aisle, because the service begins as you walk down it. Then you should remember the altar, as I shall lead you to it for the wedding prayers. Finally, you need to remember the hymn, because during that we shall go to the vestry to sign the register.' The girl was very relieved and went home feeling much happier. But imagine how the bridegroom felt on their wedding day when he heard his bride coming towards him, muttering under her breath, 'Aisle, Altar, Hymn; Aisle, Altar, Hymn'.

* * *

'Some of you may be wondering why the organ has been out of action for the last two Sundays,' said the Vicar. 'This is because of work being done to improve the instrument's facilities. When completed, our organist will be able to change his combinations without removing his hands from the keyboards.'

* * *

A Hospital Chaplain gets some odd replies to the question:
'Would you like Holy Communion?' Here are three:

  'No thanks, I'm Church of England'.
  'No thanks, I asked for Cornflakes.'
  'No thanks, I've never been circumcised.'

*   *   *

At a funeral, the relatives of the deceased chose the hymn 'Ride on, ride on in majesty'. The Vicar, intrigued by the choice, asked why this hymn had been chosen. 'Oh,' came back the reply, 'we didn't know what to have but looking through the book we saw this and thought it would be very appropriate because the deceased was a very keen cyclist.'

*   *   *

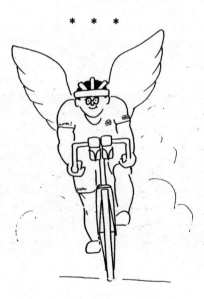

A Curate in Somerset, after baptizing a child, found himself praying that it might continue Christ's faithful Soldier and Sailor until its life's end. Not wishing to draw attention to his mistake, he let it pass. Some days later, when visiting the parents, he was asked, 'Do you know what we are going to call baby?' He replied, 'Surely, by his Christian Name.' 'Oh, no, sir, we are going to call him The Little Marine.'

* * *

Being shown round the church by the Vicar:

Visitor: 'And whose are all these names carved on this wall plaque?'

Vicar: 'It's a list of those who have died in the Services.'

Visitor: 'Prayer Book or A.S.B.?'

* * *

When the Dean retired, the Chapter asked him what he would like as a present from them all, Chapter and congregation. As he was busy reducing his library to fit the small house he was to live in, he suggested that they help him fulfil a life-long ambition to take a Mediterranean Cruise. In due course, the cruise liner set sail on a lovely day and the Dean sat in one of the deck chairs and, perhaps not surprisingly, fell asleep. Unfortunately, a fog descended on the Channel and shortly after entering the fog, the Captain ordered the fog horn and its first boom sounded out. The Dean leaped to his feet immediately and in perfect key intoned, 'O Lord, open thou our lips'.

* * *

A Vicar was having a Renewal-of-Vows Service for those who over a period of forty years or so had been joined in Holy Matrimony in the Parish Church. After the Service, during the social get-together, one couple came up to the Vicar and said, 'Oh, Vicar, thank you for inviting us today. We have so enjoyed ourselves. We want to tell you that you said something to us on our wedding day twenty years ago which we have never forgotten.' The Vicar looked suitably impressed and the lady continued: 'You said to us, "You will not remember a single word I say to you today," and, do you know, you were right!'

* * *

Vicar: 'Dost thou, in the name of this child, renounce the devil and all his works; the vain pomp and glory of the world, with all covetous desires of the same, and the carnal desires of the flesh, so that thou will not follow nor be led by them?'

Short-sighted Godparent, in stentorian tones: 'I recommend them all'.

* * *

At one Theological College, the Chapel was very small. At a certain Service, the visiting preacher, a very large Bishop, was asked to sit in a small alcove. When the Service Leader asked everyone to pray, the Bishop kneeling down brushed against all the light switches and plunged the Chapel into darkness. One of the students, opening his eyes, having closed them for the prayers, grabbed a fellow student's arm and gasped in a hoarse voice, 'My God, I've gone blind!'

* * *

A little boy was taken to his first church service, although he'd seen services on television. After it was over, his mother asked him what he'd thought of it. 'The music and the singing were all right,' he admitted, 'but I didn't think much of the news.'

* * *

'Vicar, will you pray for Annabelle next Sunday?'
'Certainly,' said the Vicar, and did so.
The following week, he said to the man, 'How is Annabelle?
Would you like me to pray for her again?'
'No thanks, Vicar, she won at 6–to–4 on.'

* * *

Newcomer to church: 'Does this church have Matins?'
Sidesman: 'Sorry, no. The Vicar's had carpets put down.'

* * *

A Vicar on the Wirral was in a most difficult situation. He had started the marriage service for a couple that regularly attended his church but he had left in the vestry the slip of paper containing their Christian Names, and he couldn't remember what they were. He hated the thought of having to ask the bridegroom his name in front of the congregation when he was supposed to know the lad well. As he ended the Preface, he did some quick thinking and produced what sounded like an authentic Prayer Book question. 'In what name comest thou to this house?' he demanded with great dignity. The Bridegroom, taken aback for a moment soon rallied: 'I come in the Name of the Father, and of the Son and of the Holy Ghost,' he replied.

* * *

In church one Sunday morning, a mother was kneeling with her small son during prayers and the boy was laughing very loudly. The mother said: 'Johnny, stop making that noise.' The little boy replied, 'It's all right, Mummy, I have just told God a joke and we are both laughing.'

* * *

A Bishop was astonished to hear little Mary say that a person must be brave these days to go to church. 'Well,' she said, 'I heard my uncle tell my aunt last Sunday that there was a canon in the pulpit, that the choir murdered the anthem and that the organist drowned the choir.'

* * *

'Name this child,' said the Vicar, as they came to the crucial part of the Baptism Service.

'Pindonim,' replied the mother.

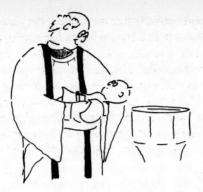

The priest was about to say the name and pour the water when it occurred to him that this was a very odd name. 'Are you sure that's what you want? Pindonim? I've never heard of it before.'

'Don't be daft,' said the mother. 'We want Albert. Look, it's pinned on 'im with a safety-pin.'

* * *

The Vicar was rather taken aback when he noticed that an old man in his congregation bowed his head every time the devil was mentioned. So he stopped him on the way out of church and asked him why he did it. The old man replied, 'Well, Vicar, a little bit of civility costs nothing and you never know!'

* * *

Parish Stewardship:

Take my silver and my gold.
Not a mite would I withhold.

But as times are rather hard,
Please accept my Barclay Card.

* * *

Moses Reid, Rector of Coppenhall from 1869 to 1880, was a noted Evangelical, and it is said that he used to ride round to pray at the farms at Rogationtide. At one farm, where the farmer was lazy, he said to his coachman, 'Drive on, John, these fields need muck not prayers.'

* * *

The small boy on his way to church for the first time was being briefed by his elder sister. 'They won't allow you to talk,' she warned him. 'Who won't?' asked the boy. 'The Hushers.'

* * *

Just outside Manchester, there is a large road sign which says, 'To the Crematorium'. Painted alongside is the slogan with the message 'Make sure the exit is clear before you enter your box'.

* * *

The Three Graces:
At Breakfast: O God, make me not like the porridge,
                  Stodgy and difficult to stir:
                  But rather like the Cornflakes,
                  Crisp and ready to serve.

At Lunch:	God bless this bunch
	As they munch their lunch.
	Give them the hunch
	To praise as they crunch.

Half-way through	
Dinner:	Praise the Lord, O my soul,
	And all that is within me
	Bless His Holy Name.

*　*　*

A story said to be going the rounds in both Australia and New Zealand concerns an Anglo-Catholic priest in the Diocese of Sydney who was taken ill suddenly. There are few of that churchmanship there and, not surprisingly, his duties had to be taken by an evangelical clergyman. The first Service was High Mass and the stand-in clergyman insisted on wearing all the usual vestments so that there would be no offence to the High Church congregation. Afterwards, he was thanked by the Churchwarden and told how well he had done. 'There is just one thing I should say in case you come again next week,' said the Warden. 'The priest here does not normally wear the book-marks as preaching bands.'

*　*　*

A very nervous Curate was conducting his first Wedding Ceremony. Despite much preparation and private rehearsal, he was horrified to hear himself saying: 'Therefore, if any man can show any just cause why they may not joyfully be loined together', and just to complete the misery of his day, when reading from the Scriptures, he managed to state that, 'The Lord is a Shoving Leopard'.

* * *

Seen in an Irish Parish Bulletin:

There will be a procession next Sunday afternoon in the grounds of the Monastery, but if it rains in the afternoon, the procession will take place in the morning.

* * *

Studdert Kennedy was very absent-minded even as a Curate in Reading. His fellow Curate, Selwyn Bean (later Archdeacon of Manchester and known as Seldom-Seen) was setting off visiting one day when a funeral cortége passed on its way to the Cemetery, the gates of which were close to the Curate's house. Selwyn Bean stopped to make sure that Studdert Kennedy, who was on duty that week, was present. Since there was no sign of him, he hurried back to his lodging, robed as quickly as possible, dashed to the head of the funeral procession and began reciting the Prayer Book words. Two days later, and in spite of a reminder, exactly the same thing happened again. Once more, an anxious Selwyn Bean rushed to the front and started the Service. This time, he heard the Cemetery Superintendent say to the Undertaker: 'Second time this week that this fool has nearly forgotten a funeral.' He says he turned to Scripture for comfort—to 1 Peter, 2, v. 20—'If when ye do well, and suffer for it, ye take it patiently, this is acceptable with God'..

* * *

Sidesman welcoming a newcomer to Church:

'Our Church is very liberal: Four Commandments and Six Do-the-best-you-can.'

* * *

From a Church Service Sheet:

Solo: Death where is thy sting?

Hymn: Search me, O God.

* * *

A deaf organ blower in a village church always continued to provide wind long after the singing of the hymns had finished. One Sunday, the exasperated organist wrote a note and asked a choirboy to give it to the blower. The choirboy, misunderstanding the organist, delivered the

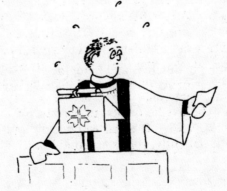

note to the Vicar, who was in the pulpit preaching. The Vicar was greatly embarrassed on reading the note which said: 'Will you, please, shut your row. People come here to hear me play not listen to your noise.'

*　*　*

She took him for better or worse, but he was worse than she took him for.

*　*　*

On the occasion of their golden wedding, the Vicar called to congratulate the late Revd. W. Muirhead-Hope and his wife, who resided in his parish. The old gentleman showed the Vicar a telegram which he had received from a friend, whose intention was to express his felicitations in the words of the twenty-third psalm. This, however, proved too much for the Post Office, which sent the message in this form: 'Surely good Mrs. Murphy shall follow thee all the days of thy life.'

*　*　*

The Annual Service for the Macclesfield and District Association of Butchers and Slaughtermen was held in the Parish Church. As they filed in, the organist was playing 'Sheep may safely graze'.

*　*　*

Announcement from the Pulpit:

Now that we have acquired an additional font, to be placed near the chancel steps, it will be possible in future to baptise babies at both ends.

* * *

'Vicar, will you pray for my floating kidneys?'

Vicar: 'I don't pray for specific complaints.'

'But you did last week, you prayed for loose livers.'

* * *

Johnny had a teddy bear with a squint. A lady asked him the teddy's name and he said, "Gladly".
   "Why do you call him Gladly?"
   "He is named after the hymn: 'Gladly my cross-eyed bear'."

* * *

One Sunday morning, in a Chapel in rural Wales, the deputising lady organist (of rather limited musical experience and ability) was frantically trying to find a suitable tune to fit the metre of an unfamiliar hymn which had been unexpectedly chosen, at short notice, by the visiting preacher. Searching through the book, she played a few bars of one after another on the old harmonium, but without success. Trying to be helpful, the Deacons, Elders and some of the congregation called out the names of tunes they thought might 'fit'. 'Try "French",' cried one. 'What's the use of that,' growled an

61

old farmer in the back pew. 'She can't even play it in Welsh.'

*　*　*

The keen evangelical group were praying for revival in their Church. 'O Lord, set this place on fire,' one man prayed fervently. Another man, kneeling beside the Vicar, muttered, 'I'm in for a thin time if God answers that.' He was an Insurance Agent.

*　*　*

A Vicar had spent some long time trying to help in a marriage breakdown. Obviously, it was not the basic cause, but the wife asserted that the rows always started over arguments as to how she should cut the bread. Her mother cut across the loaf: his mother cut down.

Some time later, speaking at a Wedding, the Vicar was trying to encourage the young couple not to let small things get out of proportion, and quoted the trouble following the insignificant matter of cutting the bread. He ended, 'So, you won't forget, will you?' and standing at the altar, with all the fervour of taking her vow, the bride said: 'Oh, I won't. I'll always buy sliced bread.'

*　*　*

An appropriate text to display on the wall of a church creche: 1 Corinthians 15. 51. 'We shall not all sleep, but we shall all be changed.'

*　*　*

Frank and Edna King called on the Vicar to arrange a Baptism. They had been richly blessed with identical twin boys. The Vicar wanted to make a special point of it and arranged that it should take place on Mothering Sunday at the Family Service, when there would be a larger than average congregation, with many children present. The Vicar tended to be of a nervous disposition and was rather anxious not to give either child the wrong name. Eventually, they arrived at the point he was dreading, when the Godmother was to hand over the first of the boys. Was it Wayne, he thought, or was it the other one? He need not have worried, for as soon as he took the babe in his arms he knew from the warm wetness on his hand that this one was Lee King.

* * *

'There will be a meeting on Wednesday evening at 7.30 to decide what colour we should whitewash the vestry, and the preacher for next Sunday will be found hanging in the porch.'

* * *

Former notice in the porch of St. Mary's, Mallenstang:

'Last out puts t'bush in t'door'.

* * *

The Chapel of Ease at Snowden Hill in South Yorkshire had a Service once a month on a Sunday afternoon. It was a room in an outhouse at a remote farm. During the war, the whole area was taken over by the U.S. Air Force and Services were suspended. When the Air Force eventually moved out, the Vicar went to reclaim possession of the premises and the Prayer Books. It was then discovered that the pages which should have been Evensong had been removed from every copy. There cannot have been a theological or liturgical reason. Matins was untouched. The solution to the mystery proved simple but surprising—MICE. The pages containing Evensong, the only Service held there, were well thumbed and greasy. That was their attraction, while Matins, presumably, only tasted of paper and print. But they had done a very neat job had those Church Mice. The U.S.A.F. was not guilty after all!

* * *

A joke about Canons: 'The bigger the gun, the bigger the bore.'

* * *

Two Cheshire farmers, one very rich and one very poor, had a very bad crop and both got into financial difficulties at the Bank. The following Sunday, they hurried to church and prayed earnestly. The poor farmer beat his breast and cried aloud, 'Lord, be merciful to me for I am a poor farmer.' Whereupon the rich farmer asked him how much he owed. '£500 would get me out of my immediate difficulties,' he replied. So, without hesitation, the rich farmer wrote him a cheque for £500 and turning, he prayed, 'Now, Lord, do you think I could have your undivided attention?'

* * *

A small girl was once asked by her mother to pray for fine weather in order that her grandmother's rheumatism might improve. When she got to her bed, the lassie knelt down and prayed: 'Oh Lord, please make it hot for Grandma.'

* * *

Little boy's prayers: 'Dear God—same as last night—Amen.'

* * *

Notice outside church:

Despite the growing inflation, the wages of sin remain absolutely the same.

* * *

RSCM report on a chorister: 'Has a very musical ear, which gives top B flat when twisted.'

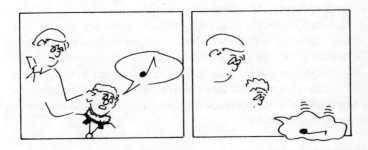

* * *

A priest in Liverpool was very much involved in the Renewal Movement. On one very hot summer evening he attended a Charismatic Prayer Meeting at a local Catholic Convent. At a particular point in the meeting, quite a few folk were praying quietly in 'Tongues'. One man, in the corner, kept repeating what sounded like the words, 'I'll have a shandy. I'll have a shandy. I'll have a shandy ...'. A friend of the priest, who obviously felt the same, spoke out—'Make that two!' It brought the house down! Was this the gift of interpretation at work?

* * *

Justice Black (U.S. Supreme Court Judge) was attending the funeral of a dignitary whom he heartily disliked and whose funeral he would not have attended had it not been expected of him. Another judge, arriving late, tiptoed into his place next to Black and whispered: 'How far has the service got?' Black whispered back: 'They've just opened for the defence.'

* * *

A visitor to an Essex church noticed a table of Kindred and Affinity pinned in the porch. Being a foreign visitor and unfamiliar with 'quaint English customs', he leaned forward to take a closer look. He began to read: 'A man may not marry his Mother, Daughter, Sister, Father's Mother, Mother's Mother' and so on. He was a little puzzled when he got to 'a man may not marry his Wife's Mother' because someone had scribbled in pencil underneath, 'Lord have mercy upon us and incline our hearts to keep this law!'

* * *

66

A young midshipman asked Nelson, on the eve of the Battle of Trafalgar, if he could offer up a prayer to God. 'Of course you can, my dear boy,' replied Nelson. The midshipman knelt on the deck and looked up to Heaven:

> 'Lord,' he said, 'I know that if it's
> your will, tomorrow we'll win this
> great battle. I also realize that
> if it's your will, the French will
> win. If you could possibly see your
> way to stay out of it altogether
> though, we'll thrash the blighters
> anyway.'

* * *

What is the difference between an Australian Wedding and an Australian Funeral?

There's one less drunk at the funeral!

* * *

Chapter 4

PULPIT RHUBARB AND BANANA-SKINS

During a rather dramatic sermon, with much gesticulating in the pulpit, a small boy whispered to his mother: 'Mummy, whatever shall we do if he gets out?'

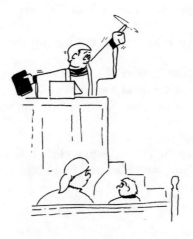

* * *

A Vicar writes:

'I was a bit put out when the Bishop of Durham was given national news coverage for saying that God is our Mother as well as our Father. I've often preached on that theme and it didn't even get into our Parish Magazine! Someone

musing on this theme re-wrote the opening verses of
Genesis:

'In the beginning God created the heaven and the earth.
And the earth was without form and void.
And darkness was upon the face of the deep.
And God said: Let there be light, and there was light.
And God hesitated and said: Could I just see the darkness
   again, please?'

* * *

With apologies to Junior School Teachers:

Two eight-year-olds were talking in the school play-
ground.
   'Do you think,' asked one, 'that thermonuclear projec-
tiles will pierce the heat barrier?'
   'No,' said the second. 'Once a force enters the substra-
tosphere . . .'
   The bell rings.
   'There goes the bell,' the first child interrupted.
   'Darn it! Now we've got to go in and string beads.'

* * *

A clergyman says that in his 'Sermon Illustration' file
there's a story filed under 'Obedience' which he hasn't
used yet. It goes like this: A woman fell down and hurt her
leg badly. She was getting on in years so her doctor
strapped up her leg, and warned her, 'Now, remember,
Mrs. Mosley, your leg will take some time to mend.
You're not to go dashing round on it. And at all costs
avoid stairs.' A month later, the doctor called to see how
she was and found that the leg had healed perfectly.

70

'Thank goodness for that,' said Mrs. Mosley. 'I felt such a fool shinning up and down the drainpipe.'

* * *

The Vicar's young son was in church and saw his father kneeling before going into the pulpit. 'What's Daddy doing?' he asked his mother. 'He's asking God to help him preach the sermon,' replied his mother. 'Why doesn't he then?' said the boy.

* * *

Going out of church one Sunday morning, a Lancashire man was greeted by his friend Joe, who had been waiting twenty minutes for him.

'Tha's late,' said Joe.

'Aye.'

'Parson bin a bit long-winded?'

'Aye.'

''appen he hasn't finished yet?'

'Oh, aye, he finished a long while sin' but he won't stop.'

* * *

'I have lost my briefcase.'

'I pity your grief.'

'It contained all my sermons.'

'I pity the thief.'

* * *

At a parish church, the Vicar was on holiday (this particular cleric was always inclined to preach over-long sermons) and the visiting priest, to the delight of the congregation, preached for eight minutes only.

When thanking this good man, the Churchwarden added: 'Your sermon was short and to the point. We all appreciated it. Our Vicar always preaches for 25–30 minutes.'

'You might have got the same from me,' replied the priest, 'but two sheets of notes fell from my desk and my little bitch chewed them up.'

'Well,' said the Warden, 'if she has pups, let me have the pick of the litter and I'll make it a present to our Vicar!'

* * *

Nervous Headboy reading a Lesson in School Assembly:

'Here beginneth the first Actor of the Chaps.'

* * *

Advice to Teacher:

'Ye ain't gotta telly, Miss? Wotever do yer do with yerself?'

'Well ... er ... friends come to call; and ... er ... I go out ...'

'Why? Don't you like 'em, Miss, them friends wot call? Can't cher afford the Licence, Miss?, 'cos you don't have to pay it, like we don't. Mi Mum says, when the fellah comes, we'll just shuv it in the cupboard!'

* * *

The Company started almost 2,000 years ago in the Middle East, trading under the Name of Joseph and Co. We were in Carpentry in a small way—Furniture, Wooden Tools, etc. When a man with the initials J.C. joined the Board, we really took off and expanded in a big way. We diversified and specialised in Life Insurance (this world and the next). We are now a Multi-national, branches in every town in the world. Most of us are in Sales.

* * *

Old lady to Vicar, who was leaving the parish:

'I am so sorry you are going. I have enjoyed your sermons so much. We never knew what sin was until you came.'

* * *

A hint that shorter sermons would be desirable and equally efficacious was suggested by a parishioner. In the course of a sermon, the Vicar had told the congregation that every blade of grass was a sermon. Passing the vicarage next morning, a gentleman, who had attended the service, saw the Vicar using the lawnmower. 'That's right, Vicar,' was the cheery greeting, 'cut your sermons short.'

* * *

School Matron to recalcitrant boarder:

'You must make your bed properly in future, Brown, or you and I will fall out!'

* * *

A Vicar was once giving a children's talk at the start of Christian Aid Week. Appropriately enough, his subject was 'Sharing God's Goodness'. To illustrate this, he had brought a packet of chocolate biscuits. Having learned that everyone would love a biscuit, he explained that as the biscuits were his, after all he had bought them, he was going to eat them all himself. Suddenly a voice from the back of the church piped up: 'You can, but you'll be sick!'

* * *

Many years ago at St. Botolph's, Cambridge, a visiting preacher was making his way to the pulpit when he slipped on the polished tiles of the Chancel, falling flat on his back. The front of the Vicar's stall, which he had reached for as he fell, came crashing down on top of him. Shaken, but unhurt, he proceeded to the pulpit. In the hymn after the sermon, the following lines were sung:

O happy servant he
In such a posture found!
He shall his Lord with rapture see,
and be with honours crowned.

* * *

The Curate was convinced of the importance of involving the congregation in the Family Service Sermon. 'Who was the funniest man in the Bible?' he asked. A teenager promptly replied, 'Samson. He brought the house down.' (We never did learn what the correct answer might be.)

* * *

The Vicar was preaching a powerful sermon concerning Death and Judgement. In the course of the sermon, he said, 'To think that all of you living in this parish will one day die.' A man in the front pew started laughing and when the Vicar sternly said, 'My good man, why do you find such a serious subject so funny?' the man replied, 'Ha! Ha! Vicar, I don't live in this parish!'

* * *

Howler from an essay:

'Vesuvius is a volcano. You can climb to the top, look over the rim and see the Creator smoking.'

* * *

The Vicar was catechizing the Kindergarten about the Christian Year. 'And what happened on Christmas Day?' he said brightly. A small boy, aged 5, replied solemnly, 'Daddy was sick on the stairs.'

* * *

A parishioner, who was never slow to complain about

anything, accosted the Vicar in the street one day. 'Just the man I want to see,' she began. 'I want you to know that I do not like the Curate's sermons.' 'But why not?' asked the clergyman. 'There are three reasons,' she said. 'First, he reads them; secondly, he reads them badly, and thirdly, they're not worth reading anyway.'

* * *

'And I have preached before royalty,' boasted the preacher. 'Only last week a man said, "If you're a preacher, I'm King Feisal of Arabia".'

* * *

A Bishop told a group of Curates the following story as a lesson in how *not* to preach. Entering a city in South America, a traveller was impressed to see a dozen targets painted on a wall, each with a bullet-hole through the exact centre of the bullseye. 'What splendid shooting,' he exclaimed. 'Who did it?' José, a boy of twelve, was pushed forward with, 'He did it, Señor.' The boy was congratulated but shook his head modestly. 'No, no, Señor. I just shoot at the walls in this town and then I paint the targets round the holes.'

* * *

Critical member of congregation to preacher who read his sermon from notes: 'If *you* can't remember it, how do you expect us to?'

* * *

The Curate during an interregnum was rather over-whelmed with the pressures of the job. On a Sunday morning, he began his sermon with an apology. 'I have been very busy this week and have not had time to prepare an address. I must therefore rely upon the promise of Scripture that the Holy Spirit will guide and direct what I say, putting the words into my mouth and moving all our hearts. Sorry about this, and I do promise to do better next week.'

* * *

It was the beginning of the season of Advent. In school, the first candle on the Advent Crown was alight when the Vicar went in to take Assembly. He asked why the candle was there and was told, 'Because it is getting near to Christmas.'

'What do you call this season before Christmas?' he asked.

At the front, one of the youngest children put up his hand and replied firmly, 'Winter.'

* * *

Reprimand from the pulpit:

'Brethren,' said the Vicar, 'you don't treat me fairly. Wait till I get a start and then if I'm not worth listening to, go off to sleep, but don't nod your heads before I get going. Give a man a chance!'

* * *

The preacher declared at the beginning of the sermon that he intended that morning to cover the whole of the Old Testament, and starting with Genesis he set out grimly to do just that. An hour and a quarter later, he was nearing the end of his task. 'Now we come to Malachi,' he declared, 'where shall we put him?' A man on the front row could stand it no longer. He rose to his feet and shouted in anger, 'Put him here; he can have my place. I'm off home.'

* * *

Part-time female required for work in the parish hall.

* * *

Two monks carrying placards—first one says, 'Drink is the enemy', the second says, 'Love your enemy'.

* * *

From a Parish Magazine:

'We would like to express our thanks to Mrs. Hill for acting as the subject during the Wolf Cubs' recent Class in First Aid and we are pleased to report that she is now out of hospital.'   Vicar.

* * *

The children were doing a Christmas version of the 'Blockbusters' Quiz during the Family Service. 'VM' was correctly identified as the Virgin Mary. 'KH' as King Herod and 'WM' as the Wise Men. 'And what,' continued a rather mindless Vicar's voice, 'was Jesus full of, beginning with G & T?'

* * *

Joseph and the Innkeeper:

A Christmas Nativity Play was arranged in a Parish of the Carlisle Diocese. The boy chosen to take the part of St. Joseph was too small for the costume so he was asked to be the Innkeeper. He did not like the change. On the night, Mary and Joseph knocked at the door of the Inn. Joseph said, 'May we come in?' The Innkeeper replied, 'Mary can but you can b . . . . . off.'

* * *

The Vicar was preaching a rousing sermon on Christian Giving, trying to persuade his rather mean parishioners to a more generous frame of mind. 'You can't take it with you,' he thundered, 'and even if you could, it would melt in the place where most of you are heading.'

* * *

'I am an atheist, thank God!'

* * *

The teachers took turns to give the lessons at Sunday

School, usually rounding them off with, 'Now, children, the moral of this story is . . .' One day, Miss Brown made the story particularly exciting and did not end it in the usual way. The children were delighted and asked if Miss Brown might not give the lesson more often. 'We like her very much,' they explained, 'because she hasn't any morals.'

*　*　*

An American Bishop told this story at a Lambeth Conference. A young priest wished to give a warning to his congregation during Advent. He did not, however, want to make it too emphatic, and so eventually his message came out as follows: 'My brethren, if we repent—more or less—and if we confess—to a certain extent—we shall be saved—as it were.'

*　*　*

There is a wall tablet to an Anglican divine of the eighteenth century which simply says, 'He preached without enthusiasm for forty years . . . of such is the Kingdom of Heaven.'

*　*　*

The definition of 'Pillars of the Church' (of which we have so many in the Church of England!): 'They hold everything up and obscure vision.'

*　*　*

There was a clergyman who regularly went into the local primary school to take a lesson. One sunny day, the children all looked particularly sleepy. To wake them up he said, 'What's grey, got a large bushy tail and eats nuts?' No one replied. He repeated the question more enthusiastically. At last, one child put his hand up and said, 'I s'pose the answer must be Jesus, but it sounds like a squirrel to me!'

* * *

How do we know that Moses wore a wig?

Because sometimes he came with Aaron and sometimes he didn't.

* * *

The man approached the Vicar at Evensong with an apology. 'I am so sorry, Vicar, I could have sworn that the sermon you preached this morning at Mattins was stolen from a book I have at home, but I was wrong, for when I got home I checked and found it was still there.'

* * *

The Vicar's wife had reached the end of her patience. The children in her Sunday School Class, one by one, wanted to leave the hall to visit the toilet. When Sunday School had ended, she gathered them all together and with clarity and emphasis she announced—'Next Sunday, everybody will go out before they come in.' (She is Irish.)

* * *

Preacher:

'This is my fourth sermon on the transforming power. Why do you look like the same old bunch?'

'My eighteenth and, ah, final point . . .'

Clergy talking:

'When I preach, I have the congregation glued to their seats.'
'Now, why didn't I think of that!'

Indefinite preaching:

'I feel I have a feeling which I feel you feel as well . . .'

Diluting the text:

A preacher describing the scene where the Philippian gaoler comes to Paul crying out, 'What must I do to be saved?' pictured Paul as answering: 'Well, what do you think?'

* * *

The Vicar had preached a long, boring sermon, made worse by the crackling from the loud speakers. At the end, he apologised with, 'There's something wrong with the microphone.' The congregation replied as one man, 'And also with you.'

* * *

A sexton is a man who minds the keys and pews.

* * *

Questions and Answers on the Bible:

Q. What does the story of the Good Samaritan teach us?
A. When I am in trouble, somebody should help me.

Q. Why did the priest in the story pass by on the other side?
A. Because the traveller had already been robbed.

Q. What do we learn from the Parable of the Lost Sheep?
A. One sinner is worth more than ninety-nine Christians.

Q. Can you find Joshua in the Book of Numbers?
A. I'll have a go if you will hand me a telephone directory.

* * *

On reaching home after the Children's Service, conducted by the Vicar, a little girl was asked how she had got on. 'Oh,' she replied, 'when Mr. —— didn't know anything, he asked us.'

* * *

At last, in the Parish of St. Ogbert-by-the-Forest, the interregnum was over and the new Vicar had arrived. The congregation listened politely to his first sermon. The following week they listened, equally politely, to his second sermon. A week later, while still listening politely to his third sermon, one or two of the congregation had a vague feeling that they had heard something similar fairly recently. During the nearly-new Vicar's fourth Sermon, some of the congregation were quite certain they had heard something similar before—it had been last week during the third Sermon. A week later, one or two people realised that the fifth Sermon was identified with the one they had heard last Sunday. After eight weeks, one brave soul asked the not-quite-so-new Vicar if he had preached that morning's sermon before. 'Yes, eight times before, to be precise,' the Vicar beamed. 'But why?' the brave soul asked, 'and when are you going to preach us a different sermon?' Again the Vicar beamed, 'When you start taking notice of the one I've preached to you eight times already,' he retorted.

* * *

If Noah had been very wise, he would have swatted those two flies!

* * *

The Vicar had a good idea for the Children's Service. He asked the children to come the following Sunday with an article that would illustrate a passage from the Bible. He was a bit disappointed with the result for only three children responded. He brought them to the front of the church. One little girl was carrying a nightdress case in the shape of a lamb.

She said, 'This reminds me that Jesus is the Lamb of God.'

'Very good,' said the Vicar. 'And what do you represent?' he asked another child who was standing with a lighted candle.

'This means that Jesus is the Light of the World,' came the reply.

The third child, a small boy puzzled him greatly. He was holding with both hands a rather large lollipop. After a lick at the lollipop, the boy said with a loud voice:

'My text is, "Hold fast to that which is good".'

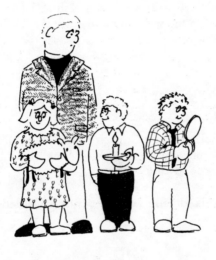

* * *

The new Vicar's sermons were carefully timed by the congregation. The first Sunday it was twenty minutes: everybody thought that was about right and they were pleased with the quality too. The next Sunday he went on for half-an-hour, but they didn't mind too much for again the quality was good. The third Sunday's sermon lasted three-quarters of an hour. This was too much and the Churchwarden complained.

'I'm so sorry,' said the Vicar, 'but it's mi teeth that's to blame.'

The Warden was baffled and waited for an explanation.

'The first Sunday was when I was wearing my new set of teeth and they were a bit uncomfortable: I had to stop after twenty minutes. By the second Sunday I had got used to them and so was able to do my usual half-an-hour.'

'So what happened today?'

'Oh, today, I was in a bit of a rush as I left the house and I picked up the wife's teeth by mistake—just couldn't get them to stop!'

* * *

During an R.E. test at a Church School, the children were asked to answer some questions by filling in the gaps. This produced the following:

'An agnostic is someone who . . . runs a Cathedral.'

* * *

There are different ways of ending a sermon. Sometimes the preacher stops without any warning at all, as if he had remembered something he has to attend to at once. Many prefer a warning that the end is in sight, rather like that given by an old Vicar in Anglesey many years ago. When the congregation saw his hands disappear under his surplice and then saw them moving about under the material, with his fingers visibly working away, they knew he was coming to the end—he was filling his pipe.

* * *

A deacon is a mass of flammable material.

* * *

In a General Knowledge Paper set at Cheltenham some thirty years ago, in a list of 'Who was?', appeared the name of Annas. The answer of one boy, who knew his facts better than his English, ran as follows:

'Annas was the High Priest decomposed by the Romans, but the Jews still called him their High Priest.'

* * *

The Hebrews had manners in the desert but didn't when they got to the Holly [sic] Land.

* * *

A howler from a school essay on classical music:

'Beethoven wrote music even though he was deaf. He was so deaf he wrote loud music.'

* * *

Children say the funniest things:

Henry VIII thought so much of Wolsey that he made him a cardigan.

The Fifth Commandment is, 'Humour thy father and mother'.

* * *

From a Parish Newsletter:

'Children are normally collected during the Offertory Hymn.'

* * *

Where in the Bible can you find adverts for Ice Cream?

'Lions of Judah' and 'Walls of Jericho'.

* * *

Who came out of the Ark fifth?

Noah's wife (Genesis 8. 15.16): 'And God spake unto Noah, saying, 'Go forth of the ark, thou and thy wife . . .'

* * *

The definition of a Rolls-Royce Preacher:

'Inaudible, well-oiled and goes on for ever.'

* * *

From a speech in the House of Commons:

'Hands off the Church of England, it's the only thing that stands between us and Christianity.'

* * *

Notice seen inside a Lincolnshire Pulpit:

'If you cannot strike oil in five minutes, stop boring.'

* * *

A Sunday School Teacher was telling the story of the Prodigal Son. 'When the son came home, the father arranged a wonderful party and expected everyone to be happy. However, there was one for whom the feast brought only great sadness. Who do you think it was?' A sad little voice said, 'Was it the fatted calf?'

* * *

Chapter 5

ECUMENICAL COCKTAIL IN THE RIGHT SPIRIT

An Englishman went to stay in New York and on his first Sunday there decided to go to church. Coming out of his hotel, he hailed a cab and said:

'Take me to Christchurch.'

'Sure,' said the Irish/American Cabbie. A few minutes later, they arrived at St. Patrick's Cathedral.

'I said Christchurch,' said the Englishman.

'Ah, sure,' said the Cabbie. 'If He's in town this morning, this is where He'll be!'

* * *

The Pope had a dream in which he was allowed to ask God three questions:

'Will there be union between us and Canterbury?' he asked.

'Not in your time,' replied God.

He tried again: 'Will women be ordained to the Catholic Priesthood?'

'Not in your time,' God answered.

Then the third question: 'Will there be another Polish Pope,' he enquired.

'Not in *my* time,' said God.

* * *

The local clergy fraternal was challenged to a new depth of friendship by one of its members.

'I think we should show our trust in one another by confessing our weaknesses and secret longings,' he said.

They agreed, and the Anglican Vicar began: 'My weakness,' he admitted, 'is drink. I have to keep a careful watch or I could become an alcoholic.'

The Roman Catholic Priest was equally frank. 'I miss female company,' he said. 'I would love to take out an attractive girl for a meal and a chat but, of course, I dare not risk it.'

The Methodist Minister was encouraged to unburden himself too. 'I'm so hard up,' he said, 'and my pay is so pathetic that there are times when I feel I would like to take twenty or thirty pounds out of the collection to buy myself a pair of shoes or something.'

By this time, a fourth member of the group was getting very agitated, shuffling his feet and glancing at his watch. 'Must go, must go,' he said, but the others insisted that before he departed he should also declare his weakness. 'Well', he said, 'since you insist. My problem is that I am a great gossip and, quite honestly, I can't wait to get out and tell all my friends the things I've just heard.'

* * *

The one-sided view:

An elderly Scottish grannie, on her way to the Kirk with her grandchildren, was passed by the Minister of another denomination riding at a canter. 'Sic a way to be riding and on the Sabbath,' she growled, and then, turning to the children, she added: "A good man is merciful to his beast" Proverbs 12, verse 10'.

Shortly afterwards, her own Minister came riding past at a gallop. 'Ah, there he goes!' said the old lady. 'The Lord bless him. Guid man! See how his heart's in his work and how eager he is to be at it. Like the Guid Book says, "Let us go speedily to pray before the Lord"; Zechariah 8, verse 21.'

* * *

Pope John XXIII was showing some of the younger Bishops around the Vatican in the early days of the great Second Vatican Council. Clearly, they were very impressed by all the great departments of State and Church Administration. 'How many people work in the Vatican, Your Holiness?' one of them asked the Pope. 'About twenty-per-cent,' came the immediate reply.

* * *

An Englishman on holiday in Glasgow goes to Hampden Park to see the local derby football match—Rangers versus Celtic. The Englishman knew that Rangers were supported by most Protestants in the City and Celtic were the Catholic side. Being an impartial spectator and all in the cause of Christian unity, he cheered loudly the good play shown by both sides in a fiercely contested first half. At half-time a Rangers' fan turned to him and said, 'Who do you think you are, a —— atheist?'

* * *

You can't be the salt of the earth without smarting someone.

* * *

An Anglican Minister, a Roman Catholic Priest and a Methodist Minister were taking a few hours off in a rowing boat. It was a hot afternoon and, resting on the oars opposite an inviting riverbank hostelry, the Anglican Minister said, 'I could certainly do with a long, cool drink,' put down the oars, stepped out of the boat and walked across the water to the other side. The Roman Catholic Priest turned to the Methodist Minister and said, 'To be sure, that's a wonderful idea. I'm ready for a drink, too,' and he also stepped out of the boat and walked across the water and joined the Anglican. The Methodist Minister called out, 'You know I don't drink but I could certainly manage a lemonade.' He stepped on to the water and disappeared with a splash. The Anglican Minister said to the Roman Catholic Priest, 'Do you think we should have told him about the stepping stones?'

* * *

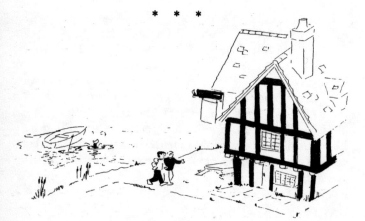

Two boys were playing in the street, one a Roman Catholic, the other a High Church Anglican. The Roman Catholic Priest came down the street and his young parishioner said, 'Good morning, Father.' A bit later, the Anglican Priest came along and the other boy called out, 'Good morning, Father,' at which the Roman Catholic boy protested. 'He's not a Father. He's got a wife and three kids!'

* * *

A Vicar of a village arranged a short service of intercession in his parish church. A few hours before it was held, he was urgently called away and invited the local Free Church Minister, with whom he was friendly, to conduct the service for him, but on condition that the minister wore a surplice, a garment to which the latter was unaccustomed. Next day, the Vicar asked him, 'Did all go well?' 'Yes,' was the reply, 'but oh! how glad I was afterwards to get my trousers on again!'

* * *

'Take things more easily,' said the Vicar, 'as the psychiatrist told the kleptomaniac.'

* * *

The old Vatican Cardinal came down to breakfast looking very haggard. He explained to his Chaplain that he had had a nightmare that had disturbed him. 'I was in the Sistine Chapel with other Bishops, planning the First Vatican Council of the 21st Century. The Pope was in the chair. One of the Bishops asked whether married Bishops would be allowed to bring their spouses to the opening service in St. Peter's. Without a moment's hesitation, the Pope replied, "But, of course, of course, how could I rule otherwise, for I certainly intend on that important occasion to have by my side my own dear husband".'

* * *

Roses are red-ish,
Violets are blue-ish.
If it wasn't for Christmas,
We'd all be Jewish.

* * *

A rabidly anti-Catholic Ulsterman was on his death bed. All the family were gathered round as he gasped: 'Fetch me a priest!' They were all thunderstruck, but his wife said to their eldest son, 'Go on, it's his dying wish. Fetch a priest.' So the son fetched a Catholic priest, who received the old man into the Church, gave him the last rites and left.

The eldest boy, with tears in his eyes, whispered to his father, 'Dad, all your life you've brought us up to believe that the Church of Rome is the anti-Christ. How came it that in your last moments you can bring yourself to join them?' With his final breath, the old man muttered, 'Better one of them beggars die than one of us!'

* * *

The local Rabbi sat next to the Vicar at the Boxing

Match. One boxer came out for the first round making the sign of the Cross over his body. The Rabbi turned to the Vicar and asked, 'Does that do any good?' The Vicar replied, 'Not if he can't box it doesn't.'

* * *

A sign supposedly seen on a farm gate:

'Trespassers may enter free. The bull will charge later.'

* * *

Rather against his better judgement, a Methodist Minister agreed to spend a day at the Races. He was thoroughly enjoying his day and was intrigued to come across the pre-race show ring. Inside was a Roman Catholic Priest, who appeared to be blessing the horses. The Methodist Minister became aware that each horse the priest blessed won its race. He decided to put a bet on the next horse the priest blessed. This he did and the race began. His horse was way out in front until the last furlong when it suddenly dropped dead. The Methodist, who was extremely annoyed, returned to the show ring and confronted the Priest. He complained bitterly, 'Every horse you blessed won, except the one I put a bet on.' 'That's the trouble with you Non-conformists,' came the reply. 'You can't tell the difference between a blessing and the last rites.'

* * *

The teacher was questioning the children about how they

had spent Christmas. One little boy described how he had opened his presents and then had gone to church with Mummy and Daddy. Another child gave details of the wonderful family party they had had. The little Jewish boy said that he too had got up early with his father, and after a hearty breakfast they had gone to the family toy factory. Hand in hand they had walked along row after row of empty shelves. 'Then Daddy sang a hymn, Miss. The one we sometimes have in school. I think it is called, "What a Friend we have in Jesus".'

* * *

Once a newly-appointed Bishop, who had an audience with the Pope, had complained that the burden of his new office had caused insomnia and he lay awake night after night suffering from great anxiety. 'Oh,' said the Holy Father, 'that's interesting. The very same thing happened to me in the first few weeks when I took over this job. Then one day my Guardian Angel appeared to me in a dream and whispered, "Giovanni, don't take yourself too seriously," and ever since then I've been able to sleep.'

* * *

'Martin Luther did not die a natural death. He was excommunicated by a bull.'

* * *

A guest at a crowded Saturday evening party was jostled and half his glass of beer landed on a Roman Catholic Priest, who had worn his clerical collar and black suit at the party. The Priest was upset, as his other suit was at the cleaners, and it seemed he would have to take services the next day smelling of beer. A helpful friend offered him some perfume. After a pause, the Priest replied, 'No thanks. The beer *I am* allowed.'

* * *

Dry-rot had devastated the parish church to such an extent that it had to be pulled down and completely rebuilt. The Vicar was comforted by the Roman Catholic Priest. He even promised a donation and, after he had consulted his lay folk, sent a donation from St. Patrick's of £250.00. 'How on earth did you get them to do it?' asked the Vicar when next they met. 'Oh, I just told them you needed money to pull down your church. They were delighted to help.'

* * *

A Methodist Minister was known to include a Prayer of Thanksgiving before his sermon every Sunday. He would thank God for the lovely flowers; for fellowship shared together; for the beautiful day; for inspiring worship, or anything else that seemed appropriate. However, there came a day in February, with snow on the ground and bitterly cold winds, when the congregation was reduced to the two stewards, who had to be there to open the premises and switch on the lights. They speculated on what the Miniser would be able to thank God for that day and thought he would find it very difficult to think of anything. But the Minister mounted the pulpit and began in his usual way. 'We do thank thee, Lord ... that we don't have many days like today.'

* * *

The Sports Editor was sent to report on the match between the Knights of St. Columba and the Free-masons, but he was not allowed to know the score because it was a secret.

* * *

'Whenever I come across a Parish Magazine, I tear it up before it can do any more damage.'   Dick Sheppard.

* * *

The friendship between Bishop David Sheppard and Archbishop Derek Worlock has been a marvellous thing for the City of Liverpool. Ecumenical relationships have improved out of recognition due in no small measure to these two men. There are many scouse stories about them, told with much affection. For instance, they are fre-quently referred to as 'Fish and Chips' for, it is said, 'They are to be taken with a pinch of salt and are never out of the papers.'

Another story concerns the day when the Archbishop took the Bishop to the top of his Cathedral to show him some of the problems they were experiencing with the roof. At one stage, both were leaning over to see more clearly a fault in the building. Far below, a passer-by grew quite alarmed as he looked up. In a loud, piercing voice he called out, 'For goodness sake don't jump. Your Giro's in the post!'

* * *

The weather was foul. Mr. O'Toole was dying. Mrs. O'Toole, turning to her daughter, said, 'Quick, run and fetch the Curate.' 'But, mother, surely you mean the Parish Priest?' 'No, I don't. What Catholic in their right mind would bring the Parish Priest out on a night like this?'

* * *

The two men met in the bar of the hovercraft that was plying between Liverpool and Dublin. One explained that he was going to the Emerald Isle for a short holiday and was looking forward to seeing something of Dublin. The other said he was on business and was in fact going for an interview for a job. He was asked for details. 'It's a j-j-job with Radio Eire. I w-w-want to be a n-n-newsreader,' he stuttered. His companion wished him the best of luck.

Fortyeight hours later, they were both back in the same place on the hovercraft, heading in the opposite direction. 'Well, come on, tell me the result. How did you get on?' 'I d-d-didn't get the job,' he said grimly. 'I should have known it would be a fix: they g-g-gave it a f-f-flippin' Catholic.'

* * *

Pope John XXIII used to say what a hard life his parents had had as small wine-growers. With a twinkle in his eye,

101

he would remark that, 'There are only three ways a man can be ruined: women, gambling and farming. My father chose the most boring of the three.'

* * *

An American visitor to a monastery guest-house in Ireland was awoken with an early morning tap on his bedroom door and the customary greeting 'Dominus Tecum' (The Lord be with you). He called out sleepily, 'Thank you, Padre, just put it down outside.'

* * *

An Anglican Archbishop and a Roman Catholic Archbishop died. When they reached the pearly gates, Peter ushered them into a Waiting Room. After they had been there an hour or two, a very pretty woman arrived and was ushered straight in. At this, their Graces protested, asking why such a youngster should get preferential treatment over men of their status. St. Peter looked at them for a moment and said, 'That young woman has just crashed her sports car which she learned to drive a year ago. In that short year she has put the fear of God into more people than your Graces have in the whole of your lives.'

* * *

At a Convent in Rome the nuns were proud of their willingness to nurse anyone of any race or creed who was in need. This was well known to the local people but they were anxious that foreign visitors to the city should be made aware of their free hospital care. They accordingly translated their aims into several foreign languages and posted them at the Convent gates. Unfortunately, their English was not as good as their medical care and their translation came out as follows:

'The nuns harbour all diseases and have no regard for religion.'

* * *

Chapter 6

ANECDOTES WITH A PINCH OF SALT

General Montgomery to his Staff Officers at a briefing:

'Now, gentlemen, as our Lord said, and in my opinion quite rightly . . .'

* * *

The galley slaves had been taught by a priest, who was one of them, to pray for relief and respite, and when this came they were overjoyed, convinced of the power of prayer. 'Men,' said the galley-master, 'you are all exhausted, I can see, but now you have a two-hour break and you will be given food and drink.' 'Hurray,' they cried, with a grateful look at the priest. 'However,' continued the galley-master, 'there is one slight snag, for this afternoon the Captain wants to go water-skiing.'

* * *

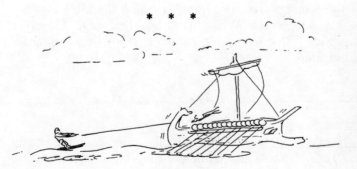

A Vicar says that when he was at school he was always first in Woodwork and Scripture and near the bottom in everything else. The Careers Master called him in to discuss his future. 'I have been looking through your reports, boy,' he said. 'Top in Woodwork and Scripture. The only job I can think of that would suit you is that of an Undertaker.'

* * *

Charles Blomfield was Bishop of Chester from 1824 to 1828 before being translated to London. It is said that while he was at Chester he sent out a directive to his clergy in rhyme. It said:

Hunt not, fish not, shoot not,
Dance not, fiddle not, flute not,
Be sure you have nothing to do with the Whigs,
But stay at home, and feed your pigs;
And above all, I make it my particular desire,
That at least once a week you will dine with the Squire.

* * *

Two young boys saw Granny reading the Bible and one said to the other, 'What on earth is she doing?' The other replied, 'Be quiet, don't disturb her: she's cramming for her finals.'

* * *

Henry Ford, on a visit to Dublin, offered a donation of £1,000 towards the building of a new hospital in the City.

The Dublin Times accidentally on purpose announced that he had promised £10,000 and praised his wonderful generosity. It was pointed out that it would look very bad if a correction had to be printed and consequently Henry Ford agreed to the larger amount. He did, however, make a condition. When the new hospital was ready, it should have an appropriate text in the entrance hall. He chose Matthew 25, V.35: 'I was a stranger and ye took me in.'

* * *

Two young married couples lived next door to one another. John was always borrowing things from his neighbour, Peter—hammer, paintbrush, lawnmower, etc., etc. It became a joke with Peter: 'Here's John. What does he want to borrow now?' Peter died suddenly. Shock! Grief! both households desolate. But, nonetheless, two days later John came round to Peter's widow: 'I shall be coming to the funeral tomorrow. Can I borrow Peter's black tie?'

* * *

At St. Andrew's in bonnie Scotland, the custom is that each player on the Old Course is announced as he steps on to the first tee. The Reverend Ian Mackenzie stepped up and was duly announced. He took an almighty swing at the ball; the club scuttled the ball through the legs of some spectators; it ran on to the 18th Green by the Clubhouse and into the hole. The voice proclaimed, 'Reverend Ian Mackenzie—Round in one!!'

* * *

The Irish Inquest Jury had debated the issue long and hard. A body had been found at the bottom of a cliff in the village. It was lunchtime and they were all hungry, so they brought in a verdict of, 'An Act of God—in suspicious circumstances'.

* * *

Proposed new terms for getting the sack

An electrician gets discharged.
A hairdresser gets distressed.
A brass player gets disbanded.
A fashion model gets defrocked.
A mathematician gets disfigured.
An artist's model gets deposed.
A civil servant gets deformed.
A Vicar gets dispirited.

* * *

The Rector was visiting a young family. The six-year-old had just returned from school.
'Good day at school, John?'
'Great! A Policeman brought his dog along.'
A lengthy and somewhat involved description of the work of a Police dog-handler ensued—to the fascination of all and especially four-year-old Rachel. The recital ended, somewhat breathlessly:
'When I grow up I want to be a Policeman.'
To which Rachel, oh-so-seriously, replied:
'And I want to be his dog!'

* * *

A Vicar was walking along the high street when he saw a man in an army greatcoat standing outside one of the main stores selling boxes of matches from a tray tied by a string around his neck. On the front of the tray hung an emotional notice: 'Please help a Veteran of the Falklands War'. The Vicar, being of a kindly disposition and wanting to help one of the lads who had braved the harsh conditions of war and climate in that far-off region of Antarctica, gave the soldier a most generous donation. The soldier, overcome by such generosity, touched his cap and said in a choking voice: 'Muchas Gratias, Señor.'

* * *

Why did God give the Irish potatoes and the Arabs oil?

Because the Irish had first choice.

* * *

A former Dean of Chester writes:

Opposite my father's old home in the village of Hartley, near Kirby Stephen, in what used to be Westmorland, there was a cottage which boasted a three-seater privy at the top of the garden. Two seats were for grown-ups while the third seat was smaller for the children.

My sisters and I delighted to hear my father tell the awful tale of how on one never-to-be-forgotten day the youngest member of the family was missing. His distracted mother and sisters searched everywhere for him, afraid that he might have fallen into the beck. At last, they heard his muffled cries. Horror of horrors, he had presumed to sit on Father's seat in the privy with disastrous consequences; the hole was too large! Clearly, he had not been listening in Sunday School or he might have remembered the prudent injunction to be content to 'sit down in the lowest seat until you are bidden to go up higher'.

* * *

The Churchwardens caught a glimpse of the Vicar in the Vestry rehearsing his sermon in front of a full-length mirror. The gestures, voice-inflections, dramatic pauses were all there. To avoid embarrassment they tip-toed away but as soon as they were out of earshot one said, "Thank goodness we've seen that, for in future we shall be able to answer the critics and say that he really does practise what he preaches."

* * *

An Archdeacon Emeritus tells this story:

I served my title in a Yorkshire mining parish—Scargill country—and I have a great regard for miners. A story I particularly like is of a Yorkshire miner who had put in a very late claim for injury at work. In Court, the Judge said to the Counsel, 'Your client is no doubt aware of Vigilantibus et non dormientibus, jura subvenient.' Counsel replied: 'In Barnsley, m'lud, they speak of little else.'

* * *

It's easy to be an angel when nobody ruffles your feathers.

* * *

The Ape House at the Zoo was treating a newcomer with a certain scepticism. 'Who are you?' asked one of the Chimps. 'Well, according to Darwin,' replied the new ape, 'I'm my keeper's brother.'

* * *

The Vicar had given a lesson in school on the Ten Commandments. Now came the time to discover whether the children were able to apply them to their everyday lives.
"If I take a five-pound note out of a man's pocket who is standing in front of me in a queue which Commandment have I broken?"
"Please Sir, the eighth, which says 'Thou shalt not steal'."
"Well done. Now for a more difficult question. If I pull off the cat's tail from its body, which Commandment have I broken then?"
There was a long thoughtful silence and then one little boy decided to try his luck.
"Please Sir, is it the one that says, 'What God has joined together let no one put asunder'?"

* * *

A well-authenticated story tells us that in 1741 Handel was on his way to Dublin from London and was held up in Chester because of strong winds; eventually setting sail from Parkgate in Wirral. He wanted to try out some parts of his new Oratorio 'Messiah' so he engaged one of

Chester Cathedral Lay Clerks, a man named Janson, who apparently failed to please the great composer with his singing. Handel is reported to have shouted at him, 'You scoundrel! Did you not tell me that you could sing at sight?' To which the meek reply from the intimidated singer was, 'Yes, sir, but not at *first* sight!'

* * *

A baby mouse saw a bat for the first time in its life and ran home screaming to its mother saying it had just seen an angel.

* * *

A young lad came downstairs and asked his Dad: 'Is it true, Dad, from dust we came and to dust we return?' His father replied, 'Yes, that is quite right.' The boy said, 'Well, do you mind coming upstairs and looking under my bed because I am not quite sure whether somebody is coming or going.'

* * *

The Chairman and Secretary of the local Communist Party were interviewing an applicant for a key party post. The Chairman asked him, 'If you had two houses, what would you do?' He answered: 'I would sell one and give the money to the Party.' The second question came from the Secretary: 'If you owned two cars, what would you do?'. 'Sell one, and give the money to the Party.' All seemed very promising. The Chairman put his last question: 'Suppose you had two bicycles, what would you do?'

The applicant turned bright red with rage and stormed out of the room without answering. Surprised, the Chairman asked the Secretary: 'Why do you think he did that?' 'Ah, you see,' replied the Secretary, 'he's *got* two bicycles.'

*   *   *

A little boy, after attending a lesson at school on human origins, was asked to write an essay on the subject 'How life begins'.

At tea-time the same evening, he asked his mother how he had come to be born. His mother replied that he had been found under a gooseberry bush.

'What about Dad?' the little boy asked.

'He came from a gooseberry bush too,' said Mum. 'And Grandad?' asked the boy, (dreading the answer) 'where did he come from?'

'Oh, the same,' said Mum, 'he came from a gooseberry bush too.'

After tea, the boy began his essay: 'According to my Mum, there hasn't been a normal birth in our family for the past three generations.'

*   *   *

Did you hear about the dog that visited a flea circus and stole the show?

*   *   *

The Vicar enjoyed a turn of speed and one dark and stormy night was belting down the M6 when he heard a tapping noise on the side window of his car. Peering through the rain and murk, he saw a helmeted head the other side of the glass, and taking a closer look saw a motor-cyclist alongside, keeping up with his car. The motor-cyclist was standing up, one foot on the saddle and the other foot on the handlebars doing the steering. As the tapping continued, the Vicar wound down the window and saw the motor-cyclist with a cigarette in his mouth and heard him say: 'Got a light, mate?' By now, the Vicar was so bemused that he handed his lighter through the window and said: 'Don't you know you could kill yourself doing that?' The motor-cyclist answered, 'Yes, that's what they all say, but I am down to three a day.'

* * *

An academic approach:

If you borrow from one author, it's plagiarism.
If you borrow from many authors, it's research.
If we steal thoughts from the moderns, it would also be cried down as plagiarism; if from the ancients, it would be cried up as erudition.

* * *

An old lady had always used a paraffin lamp. The local Council insisted on converting the house to electricity. The first electricity bill came to 28p. She showed it to the Vicar when he visited. He was quite concerned and asked whether she knew how to use electricity properly. 'Oh, yes,' she said. She thought it was wonderful. She switched on the light every night so she could see to light her paraffin lamp!

* * *

Dear Paddy,

The Vicar here thinks very highly of your father. He's given him a job so important that he has five hundred men under him. He's cutting grass in the churchyard.

* * *

Test for an Irish ordinand:

Q. What do you know about Damascus?
A. Kills all known germs, dead!

Q. Who was born in a stable?
A. Red Rum.

Q. How did David kill Goliath?
A. With the Acts of the Apostles.

Q. Who was Noah's wife?
A. Joan of Arc.

Q. What is Copper Nitrate?
A. A policeman's overtime.

* * *

A man decided to commit suicide and climbed to the top of a high building in Manchester, intending to throw himself down. A local Vicar was sent up to try to talk him out of it. The following conversation ensued:-

Vicar: 'Don't jump. It's a lovely day.'
Man: 'I don't care.'

Vicar: 'Think of the wife.'
Man: 'I'm not married.'
Vicar: 'What about the girl friend?'
Man: 'It's all over.'
Vicar (desperately): 'Manchester United are playing at home today.'
Man: 'I support City.'
Vicar: 'Well, perhaps you had better jump!'

* * *

In the U.S.A. it has been suggested that in laboratory experiments T.V. Evangelists should be used instead of rats. The reason is twofold: First, there are more of them; and secondly, there is less emotional attachment.

* * *

'You mustn't pull the cat's tail.'
'I'm only holding it—the cat's pulling.'

* * *

A woman telephoned her Bank and spoke to the Accountant who looked after her holdings. 'I want to make some changes,' she said. The Accountant asked for more details. 'Are you interested in Conversion or Redemption?' he asked. 'Good heavens!' came the reply. 'I must have got the wrong number. I wanted the Bank of England not the Church of England.'

* * *

It was Christmas Day. The children woke up to see their Christmas presents. The two boys had presents that looked identical. The first boy opened his. He was not pleased. It was a bucket of manure. He cried and sulked. Meanwhile, the second boy opened his. 'Yippie!' he said, 'it's a bucket of manure.' The first boy said, 'I don't see what's so good about a bucket of manure,' to which the second boy replied: 'Don't you see, there must be a horse round here somewhere.'

* * *

Sitting down to the meal at one of those big 'Family' occasions, a priest found himself across the table from his brother's most recent foster child. It was the first time they had met each other and he could see that the little girl was mesmerised by the dog-collar. Her curiosity exploded just at the same time as there was one of those awkward lulls in conversation around the table, and a shrill little voice rang clearly, 'Has he broken 'is neck then?'

* * *

Interviewer at front door: 'I am conducting a survey. Would you mind telling me if you have a bidet?'
Householder: 'No, we haven't. We're Church of England.'

* * *

Three Scotsmen attended church one morning. When the

collection plate was handed round, one of them fainted and the other two carried him out.

* * *

The most successful businessman the world has ever known was Noah. He floated a successful company while the rest of the world was going into liquidation.

* * *

I am a sundial
And I make a botch
Of what is done much better
By a watch.   [Sundial in Dorset]

* * *

A story to comfort the clergy who have difficulty remembering names.

Sir Thomas Beecham, returning to his hotel room in Manchester after conducting a concert at the Free Trade Hall, was keen to mount the staircase and return to his room. In the foyer, however, he noticed a distinguished-looking woman, whom he vaguely recognised but could not place in his memory. She saw him, so he paused for a few words. In the course of the brief chat, he remembered that she had a brother and, hoping this might identify her, he asked how her brother was and if he was still in the same job. 'Oh, he's quite well,' the lady replied, 'and he's still the King.'

* * *

Sir Edwin Lutyens to hotel waiter:
  'What is this?'
  'Cod, sir.'
  'Cod! Then it must be that piece of cod that passeth all understanding.'

* * *

A large American saloon car pulled up outside the parish church. The old Verger was busy cutting the grass. The car window slid down and a voice with a strong American accent called: 'Say, any great men born around these parts?' 'Nope,' came the reply, 'only babies!'

* * *

The road to the local Crematorium ran through the golf course just outside a town where a Cheshire Vicar lived some years ago. It was the custom for players to pause, remove caps and stand with heads bowed whenever a cortége wound its way across the course. Everyone adhered to this respectful custom except the Vicar's partner, Raymond. He never allowed anything to inter-rupt their regular Friday morning engagement. You can imagine the Vicar's astonishment when one Friday, as Raymond was preparing for a vital putt on the final green, he suddenly stopped, removed his cap and stood reverently while a funeral passed along the road. The

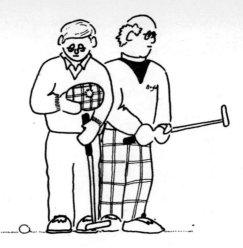

Vicar expressed surprise at this unusual mark of respect.
'Ah, well,' replied Raymond, 'I feel it's the least I could
do for she has been a splendid wife for the past forty
years.'

* * *

One night, Albert went to his favourite local on his bike
and thoroughly enjoyed having a drink and meeting his
friends. It was only when he was back home having
supper that he realised he had walked home and left his
bike propped up outside the pub. His wife was very
pessimistic. 'You haven't a lock on it and it's nearly new;
somebody will have pinched it by now, you can be sure.'
But Albert was already on his way, and he was breathless
but greatly relieved to find on his arrival that his bike was
still leaning against the wall. He started to ride home in a
very happy frame of mind. His musings turned theological as he thanked God for his good fortune. He felt he
should do something about it and since he had to pass the

church on route, he knew what he wanted to do. He stopped outside and found a fiver in his pocket: quietly opening the door, he entered into the darkness: knelt for a moment to express his gratitude, and feeling his way to the offertory box, he popped in the money. Felt better for it too, that is, until he came out and found somebody had stolen his bike!

* * *

'On reaching the age of 90, Members of St. Mary's Mothers' Union Branch will no longer pay subscriptions but will become Life Members.' [From a Parish Magazine]

* * *

Chapter 7

GOOD WINE KEPT UNTIL THE END

Did you hear the story of St. Peter at the Pearly Gates checking on newcomers? 'Who is there?' he cried as a figure approached.

'It is I,' was the reply.

'Another pedantic, boring teacher!' said St. Peter.

* * *

A Vicar decided to photograph the ghost that haunted his church. This would convince the doubters. He even asked permission from the ghost itself. Then came the great day when, with all the equipment at the ready, he prepared

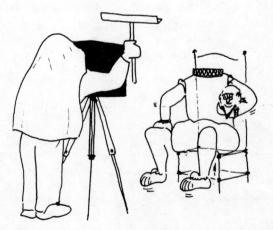

for action. The ghost appeared. The Vicar pressed the switch . . . nothing happened. Alas, 'The spirit was willing but the flash was weak.'

* * *

Rhyme and Reason:
> If your nose is close to the grindstone
> And you hold it there long enough,
> In time you'll say there's no such thing
> As brooks that babble and birds that sing.
> These three will all your world compose
> Just you, the stone and your poor old nose.

[200-year-old stone in a country cemetery]

* * *

A parishioner had buried his wife after thirty years of happy married life. He had her headstone engraved: 'The light of my life has gone out.' A few years later, he remarried and the original inscription on the gravestone of his first wife now read: 'The light of my life has gone out, but I have struck another match.'

* * *

Inscription on the gravestone of a hypochondriac:

'See, I really was ill!'

* * *

124

One day, a man arrived at the gates of Heaven, where he was greeted by St. Peter, who asked him a number of questions about his life on earth. Among these, he asked whether he'd had any interesting hobbies. The man replied that he'd been an international Rugby referee. Later, St. Peter asked if he'd done anything heroic during the course of his life. The man replied, 'I was refereeing the England versus Wales match at Cardiff Arms Park. The result would determine who won the Five-Nation Championship and the Triple Crown. Wales were winning 18–16 and in the final minute I awarded England a penalty right in front of the Welsh posts.' 'That's very interesting,' said St. Peter, as he searched through his files, 'but I can't seem to find any record of that here. When did it happen?' 'About five minutes ago,' the man replied.

* * *

The one comment that has remained with a certain priest over the years was the reaction of a Churchwarden when the Council was asked to make the Church Hall available for the use of non-Church activities in the parish—'Anyone would think we were a Charitable Organisation!'

* * *

Woman to Dr. Johnson: 'Thank goodness you have missed out all the naughty words from your Dictionary.' Dr. Johnson: 'Ah, then you have looked for them!'

* * *

When the new Church of St. Mary the Virgin was to be

consecrated, the Vicar was invited by a close friend to choose from his Collection of relics. The Vicar, much moved by this offer, hurried off to make his choice, and we, the staff, waited expectantly for such a treasure to be brought back. In walked the Vicar carrying a box covered with a purple cloth. 'It came down to choosing between a piece of the Table of the Last Supper or a piece of St. Peter's chains,' reported the Vicar, 'and I've brought the Table of the Last Supper.' There was awed silence. 'Why did you choose this and not the other?' he was asked innocently. 'Well,' he said, 'the other seemed so far-fetched!'

* * *

What did Jonah do for three days in the belly of the big fish?

Sang, of course, for everybody sings in Wales, boyo!

* * *

Heaven is an English house, an American salary, a Chinese cook and a Japanese wife.

Hell is a Japanese house, a Chinese salary, an English Cook and an American wife!

* * *

The economic policy of the large fish in the Book of Jonah:

'Small profits/prophets and quick returns!'

* * *

Small boy: 'Grandfather, were you in the Ark?'
Grandfather (very grumpy): 'No, I was *not* in the Ark.'
Small boy (with relentless logic): 'Well, why weren't you
drowned then?'

* * *

Don't worry! You will either be well or you will be ill. If
you are well, you have nothing to worry about, and if you
are ill, only two things can happen—you will either get
better or you will die. If you get better, you have nothing
to worry about, and if you die, only two things can
happen. You will either go to heaven or you will go to
hell. If you go to heaven, you have nothing to worry
about, and if you go to hell, you will be so busy shaking
hands with all your friends, you won't have time to worry!

* * *

How did the people of Paris find Quasimodo?

'They followed a hunch.'

* * *

An old woman, whose reputation was far from good, was
seriously ill and was being visited by the Vicar. He
warned her of the outer darkness, where there would be

'weeping and gnashing of teeth'. Dropping his voice to a solemn tone, he repeated, 'weeping and gnashing of teeth'. With a defiant but toothless grin, the old lady retorted: 'Let them gnash 'em as 'as 'em!'

* * *

And now let us pray for those who are sick of this parish.

* * *

A Painter and Decorator, not noted for his honesty, watered down his paint but charged his customers for the full quantity. On one occasion, the finished result looked so bad that he feared he would be found out. 'What can I do now?' he wailed. From the heavens a great voice cried out, 'Repaint! Repaint! and thin so more!'

* * *

'What sort of lighting did Noah have on the ark?'

'No, not arc lighting—It was flood lighting.'

* * *

A man taking a short cut through a churchyard in the dark fell into a deep grave which had been prepared for the next day's funeral. Try as he would, the sides were so steep he couldn't get out, and he sank back exhausted. Sometime later, another man crossed the same churchyard and he too fell in. Thinking himself alone and frightened, he struggled to grapple up the sides. The first man leant forward, touched him on the shoulder and said, 'Son, you won't get out of here!' But, oh boy, he did!

* * *

The trouble with temptation is—it's so often gift-wrapped.

* * *

Two brothers died at the same time and arrived at the Pearly gates together, where they were interviewed by St. Peter. He said to the first brother, 'Have you been good during your life on earth?' and he replied, 'Oh, yes, your saintliness, I've been honest, sober and industrious, and I've never messed around with women.' 'Good lad,' said St. Peter and gave him a beautiful, gleaming white Rolls-Royce. 'There's your reward for being a good boy.' Then he said to the other brother: 'And what about you?' He said, 'Well, I've always been very different from my brother. I've been crooked, drunk, idle and a devil with the women.' 'Ah well,' said St. Peter, 'boys will be boys and at least you've owned up to it. You can have this,' and he gave him the keys to a Mini.

The two brothers were about to get in their cars when the one who'd been naughty started roaring with laughter. The other one said, 'What's so funny then?' He said, 'I've just seen the Vicar riding a bike!'

* * *

Dai Jones, Welsh International, playing on the wing for Wales, scored a winning try against England but the ball was a forward pass. In the Dressing Room, he confessed this to his fellow Welshmen, who all told him not to worry as it was definitely *not* a forward pass. In Chapel on the following Sunday, he told all the deacons that the ball was forward. They assured him that the ball certainly was not forward. All through his life Dai carried this heavy load of guilt and eventually he died. He got to the pearly gates and thought that the best thing to do was to confess straight away. He said, 'I'm Dai Jones, Welsh International, played on the wing for Wales against England, scored the winning try but the ball was a forward pass.' A voice said, 'Certainly not. It was not a forward pass.' 'Oh, it was,' Dai said, 'I know. I have lived with this all my life and I can't stand it any more.' The voice again reassured him. 'You must take my word for it. Now come into heaven and welcome.' 'I feel better for the first time for years,' said Dai. 'Thank you, St. Peter.' The voice interrupted with, 'Oh, I'm not St. Peter. It's his day off. I'm St. David.'

* * *

A Vicar was leaving his parish after a long incumbency. At the Valedictory Service, he boasted in his final sermon that he was very happy leaving the parish without a single enemy. After the service, a parishioner asked him, 'Vicar, how can you say so emphatically that you are leaving the parish without a single enemy?' The Vicar replied, 'I have buried them all!'

* * *

'How do you reconcile St. Matthew's version of our Lord's words—"Are not two sparrows sold for a farthing?"—with St. Luke's—"Are not five sparrows sold for two farthings?",' once asked a seeker after the truth. There was a decided twinkle in the eyes of the clergyman as he replied: 'Because you get them cheaper if you take a quantity.'

* * *

'It will be of great assistance if parishioners will attend to their own graves.'   [From a Parish Magazine]

* * *

A man met a friend in the street whom he hadn't seen in years. 'And how's your dear wife?' he asked. 'She's gone to heaven,' was the reply. 'Oh, I'm so sorry,' said the first man. He quickly realised that that didn't sound right so he corrected himself: 'I mean, I'm glad.' That was even worse. He made a third attempt: 'I mean, I'm surprised.'

* * *

Epitaph for a Dentist:

> Stranger beware and tread with gravity:
> Here lies John Smith filling his last cavity.

* * *

> Here lie I near the vestry door;
> Here lie I because I was poor;
> The further in the more you pay;
> Here lie I as warm as they.

* * *

> Here lies the Reverend Donald MacIntyre,
> Scottish Missionary;
> Accidentally shot by his native bearer
> whilst on a missionary journey in the jungle.

'Well done, thou good and faithful servant'.

* * *

The Vicar died and went to heaven. He was a bit disappointed to find that he had to undergo a period of penance. This consisted of being shackled to an old rag-bag of a woman whom he had to drag round with him wherever he went. After a few days of this he came across his former bishop and was full of envy when he saw that he was shackled to a very attractive young lady, a real dolly-bird. He made his way to the office to complain to St. Peter. He received short shrift and got the curt reply, "This has nothing to do with you. You get on with your penance and allow that young lady to get on with hers."

I have no relish for the country; It is a kind of healthy grave.

I never read a book before reviewing it; it prejudices a man so.

(Rev. Sydney Smith, 1771–1845)

*   *   *

Man's life is like unto a winter's day,
Some break their fast and so depart away,
Others stay dinner then depart full fed;
The longest age but sups and goes to bed.
Oh, reader, then behold and see,
As we are now, so must you be.

[Epitaph written by Bishop Henshaw]

*   *   *

Here lies a learned Divine;
He died in a fit
Through drinking Port Wine. 1828.

*   *   *

On the death of his wife, a man telephoned the local florist for a wreath. 'What wording would you like on the ribbon?' asked the assistant. 'I'd like REST IN PEACE on one side,' said the man, 'and WE SHALL MEET IN HEAVEN on the other side, if there's room.' When the wreath was delivered, the ribbon bore the message:

REST IN PEACE ON ONE SIDE AND WE SHALL

MEET IN HEAVEN ON THE OTHER SIDE IF
THERE IS ROOM.

* * *

He first deceased: she for a little tried
To live without him, liked if not, and died.
[Sir Henry Wotton]

* * *

On Sunday, a father and his small daughter walked
slowly home through the churchyard looking at the
headstone inscriptions on their way. Suddenly, the girl
shouted excitedly, 'Daddy, come and look. I think I've
found a live one.' Hurrying over, the father found his
daughter gazing wide-eyed at a headstone bearing the
legend, 'She is not dead but sleepeth'.

* * *

Peas to his Hashes.

[Epitaph on a London Cook]

* * *

Here lies Anne Mann;
She lived an old maid and died an old Mann.

[Epitaph from Devonshire]

* * *

Johnny would not eat his prunes. His parents were very cross and eventually banished him to his bedroom with the comment that not only they were cross but God was cross as well. Shortly after this domestic incident, a thunder-storm blew up and mother became anxious for her little boy, but father insisted he stay where he was and take his punishment. However, when the house next door was struck by lightning mother could stand it no longer and flew upstairs to her son's room. At first she couldn't see him, but finally spied him kneeling by the window looking out. She was just in time to hear him say calmly, 'How ridiculous, God, all this fuss over four prunes.'

* * *

Do you ever wonder how many fig leaves Eve tried on before she said, 'I'll take this one'?

* * *

Nothing is more responsible for the good old days than a bad memory.

* * *

The last waltz at the Annual Dinner Dance for the Union of Spiritualist Mediums was entitled, 'I'll see you again'.

* * *

Where there's a will there's relations.

* * *

Some people bring happiness wherever they go, and some people bring happiness whenever they go.

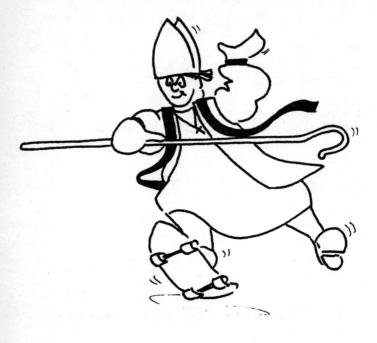

* * *

'To everything there is a season, and a time to every purpose under the heaven: A time to weep, and a time to laugh . . .'

[Ecclesiastes 3:1&4]

INDEX

138

139